Antimicrobial Resistance and Control

Azhar ul Haque Sario

Copyright

First Printing, 2025

Azhar.sario@hotmail.co.uk

ORCID: https://orcid.org/0009-0004-8629-830X
Disclaimer: This book is free from AI use. The cover was designed in Microsoft Publisher

Contents

Unveiling the Silent Pandemic

The Unseen War: Beyond the Superbug Headlines

We hear a lot about "superbugs," those headline-grabbing bacteria that shrug off our best antibiotics. They're the villains we know, like MRSA or the terrifying "nightmare bacteria" haunting hospital wards. And they are terrifying, stealing lives – over a million worldwide each year directly linked to their resistance. They turn routine infections into deadly gambles and cast a long shadow over surgeries, cancer treatments, even childbirth. The progress medicine has gifted us feels suddenly fragile.

But this fight is bigger, deeper, and quieter than just bacteria. Imagine antimicrobial resistance not as a single monster, but as a rising tide, or perhaps an invisible enemy adapting on multiple fronts simultaneously. While we've been laser-focused on bacteria, other microscopic threats have been learning our tricks, evolving their own defenses.

Meet the Silent Saboteurs:

The Ghostly Fungus: Lurking in the corners, especially in hospitals, is a relatively new menace: Candida auris. Think of it as a fungal ghost – hard to identify, stubbornly resistant to multiple antifungal drugs, and clinging invisibly to surfaces, ready to prey on the weakest among us. It spreads silently, causing devastating outbreaks and reminding us that the fungal kingdom is also fighting back, with mortality rates in vulnerable patients painting a grim picture. It's a chilling whisper of a threat that's rapidly finding its voice.

The Viral Shape-Shifters: Viruses, masters of adaptation, aren't sitting idle either. Remember the yearly scramble for a new flu shot? That's partly because the influenza virus constantly tweaks its armor against antiviral drugs like Tamiflu. HIV, the virus we've fought so hard to control with life-saving antiretrovirals, learns to dodge these treatments too, threatening to unravel years of progress for individuals. Even newer victories, like cures for Hepatitis C, face the potential shadow of resistance. Our antiviral shields are being tested, constantly.

The Persistent Parasites: In vast swathes of the world, the battle against ancient parasitic diseases is hitting a dangerous snag. Malaria, particularly the deadly Plasmodium falciparum, is developing resistance to our front-line treatments (ACTs). This resistance, spreading like a stain across maps in Asia and now appearing in Africa, means treatments take longer to work, giving the parasite more time to harm and spread. It threatens to roll back decades of hard-won gains. Similarly, tiny worms causing neglected tropical diseases are also learning to survive treatments, keeping millions trapped in cycles of poverty and illness.

Connecting the Dots: A Battle on All Fronts

This isn't just a collection of separate problems; it's a tangled web. The rise of resistance across bacteria, fungi, viruses, and parasites puts everything at risk. The safety net we rely on for C-sections, hip replacements, chemotherapy, organ transplants – it's fraying because the infections we need to prevent or treat are becoming harder to defeat.

So, how do we fight an enemy with so many faces? We need to stop looking at the battlefield through narrow keyholes.

Imagine this: A hospital ICU is suddenly seeing more drug-resistant TB and more Candida auris infections. Instead of two separate alarms, an integrated "threat radar" lights up. Doctors and infection control teams can now ask: What links these? Is there a shared vulnerability in our patients? A lapse in cleaning protocols that allows both an airborne bacterium and a surface-clinging fungus to thrive?

This "connecting-the-dots" approach is crucial. By tracking resistance across all types of microbes together, we can:

Spot hidden connections: Understand shared risks and weaknesses in our defenses.

Mount a smarter defense: Implement broader infection control measures that tackle multiple threats at once.

Use resources wisely: Focus screening and interventions where they're needed most.

Truly grasp the danger: Understand the devastating impact when vulnerable patients face multiple resistant infections.

This multi-pronged resistance is more than a scientific challenge; it's a fundamental threat to human health and the marvels of modern medicine. We need to see the whole picture, understand the interconnectedness, and build a unified shield against this pervasive, shape-shifting war. The future of medicine may depend on it.

The Shadow Epidemic: How Superbugs Target Our Most Cherished and Overlooked

Forget the sterile labs and global infection maps for a heartbeat. Let's talk about us. Let's talk about the way antimicrobial resistance – the terrifying rise of "superbugs" that shrug off our medicines – isn't just a vague, hovering threat. It's a predator. And like any predator, it stalks the vulnerable, sinking its teeth deepest where defenses are already worn thin. This isn't an equal-opportunity crisis. It casts a chilling shadow, longest and darkest, over the cradles holding our newest lives, the chairs holding our elders, and the communities fighting hardest just to get by. It's a story written not just in Petri dishes, but in worried whispers, in shortened lifespans, and in the quiet desperation of inequality.

First Breaths, First Battles: Our Children on the Front Lines

Imagine the miracle of a newborn's first cry – a sound bursting with promise. Now imagine that promise being immediately threatened because the simplest infection, one that should be easily treatable, has become a monster. For infants, especially those born too soon or in places where resources are scarce, their brand-new immune systems are like tiny, untested shields. They rely on antibiotics, sometimes for sheer survival. Yet, this very reliance makes them ground zero for resistance.

Think of neonatal sepsis, a terrifying firestorm in a tiny body. Around the world, especially within the sterile walls of Neonatal Intensive Care Units (NICUs), doctors whisper about first-choice antibiotics failing more and more often. Picture parents watching their impossibly small child fight not just prematurity or illness, but an infection caused by bacteria that have learned to outsmart our cures. The numbers are staggering – hundreds of thousands of newborn lives lost each year because the medicines didn't work. Clinicians are forced onto a knife's edge, needing to use bigger, potentially harsher "last-resort" drugs (if they even have them), adding risk upon risk. And where poverty casts its own shadow, malnutrition weakens these tiny fighters further, making them more susceptible to infection, and thus, more exposed to the drugs that might be failing them.

Hope in Action: But even here, humanity fights back. Picture NICUs transforming into fortresses of care – using lightning-fast tests to identify the exact bacterial enemy and its weaknesses, allowing for targeted strikes instead of hopeful guesses. Imagine the simple, powerful rhythm of constant handwashing, the meticulous cleaning, the careful separation of sick infants – acts of profound care, like those in a South African unit, proving that even the most dangerous superbugs can be contained with vigilance and dedication.

The Golden Years Under Siege: Our Elders Facing Compounded Risks

Years grant us wrinkles, wisdom, and stories etched into our faces. But time also gently lowers our body's natural defenses. This "immunosenescence," combined with the chronic conditions many elders live with – the diabetes, the heart disease, the breathing troubles – creates a unique vulnerability. Every necessary hospital visit, every trip to the clinic, even residing in a long-term care facility, becomes an unintentional roll of the dice, increasing the odds of encountering bacteria that have learned to cheat death.

Think of your grandmother battling pneumonia that just won't quit, or a persistent urinary tract infection (UTI) that laughs off standard treatments. These aren't just inconveniences; they're serious threats. For older adults, infections caused by resistant bacteria mean longer, more draining hospital stays, higher chances the treatment won't work, a greater risk of devastating complications, and a tragically increased chance that this infection will be their last. Across Europe, the sobering reality is that the majority of lives claimed by AMR belong to those over 65.

Hope in Action: Protecting this generation means defending the places they call home. Envision long-term care facilities where staff are champions of hygiene, meticulously trained to prevent infections spread through touch or devices like catheters. Picture thoughtful "antibiotic stewardship," where prescriptions are questioned, ensuring they're truly necessary, perfectly targeted, and stopped promptly. Imagine facilities screening residents for hidden resistant bugs to prevent silent spread, and the simple, powerful protection offered by flu and pneumonia vaccines, stopping infections before they ever demand an antibiotic.

The Vicious Cycle: Where Poverty and Resistance Collide

Poverty isn't just about empty pockets; it's about empty defenses. In communities wrestling with unsafe water, inadequate sanitation, and poor nutrition, infections find fertile ground. More infections inevitably mean more antibiotic use, often without a doctor's guidance, sometimes with drugs bought informally, their quality unknown.

Imagine the cruel irony: needing medicine desperately, only to receive a counterfeit or substandard antibiotic, one too weak to cure but strong enough to teach the bacteria how to survive the real thing next time. It's a devastating feedback loop: lack of basic needs fuels infection, infection fuels demand for often inappropriate or fake antibiotics, which fuels resistance, making future infections deadlier and harder to escape. In the chaotic landscapes of conflict zones or the dense humanity of refugee camps, this cycle spins into a terrifying vortex. Overcrowding, broken sanitation, shattered healthcare, and high rates of injury create a perfect storm for untreatable infections to rage, often met only with best-guess treatments because diagnostic tools are a luxury.

Hope in Action: Even in the most challenging circumstances, resilience finds a way. Picture humanitarian groups like MSF in places like Cox's Bazar, fighting AMR not just with medicine, but with clean water projects, latrine construction, and hygiene education – the fundamental building blocks of health. It looks like intense efforts to secure quality-assured medicines, training local health workers in the precious art of rational prescribing, and setting up surveillance, however basic, to understand the enemy they face. On a larger scale, it demands dismantling the deadly trade in fake drugs, building accessible clinics, and investing in the infrastructure that allows communities to break free from the grip of infection and resistance.

Conclusion: A Fight for Fairness

Antimicrobial resistance is more than a scientific puzzle; it's a profound question of fairness. Its reflection looks different depending on who it touches: the fragile infant in an incubator, the revered elder in their favorite chair, the resilient family in a struggling community. The superbug crisis speaks the language of inequality, hitting hardest where life is already precarious.

Acknowledging this isn't just data analysis; it's the very soul of the solution. We cannot conquer this threat with blanket strategies. We must walk onto the specific battlegrounds where the fight is fiercest – from the high-tech NICU to the refugee camp relying on basic hygiene. We must tailor our weapons, reinforce the weakest points in our collective human defense. To turn away from the disproportionate suffering of our children, our elders, and those trapped by poverty is not just strategic folly – it's a betrayal of our shared humanity. Protecting them is protecting the future, ensuring this silent pandemic doesn't get the last word in their stories, or ours.

The Invisible Shapeshifters: Witnessing Evolution on Fast-Forward

Antibiotic resistance isn't just a problem; it's a living, breathing crisis authored by evolution itself. We're talking about microscopic adversaries – bacteria – that are masters of adaptation, rewriting their own rulebooks at lightning speed to defy the very medicines we created to control them. For too long, we've been like historians, documenting resistance after the battle was lost. But the game is changing. We're becoming war correspondents, embedded on the front lines, using bleeding-edge technology to watch the enemy adapt as it happens.

Imagine tiny organisms, invisible to the naked eye, engaged in a desperate arms race against us. Their secret weapon? Evolution on overdrive. Sometimes, it's a lucky typo – a random mutation in their DNA – that accidentally makes them invisible to an antibiotic's attack or gives them stronger shields to deflect the blow. Think of it as a spur-of-the-moment disguise that suddenly works.

But their real genius lies in their ability to cheat. Bacteria are incredibly social (in a purely genetic sense!). They don't just rely on slow, generational change. They pass cheat sheets – snippets of DNA carrying resistance instructions – between themselves like contraband notes in a classroom. This "horizontal gene transfer," often using tiny, mobile vehicles like plasmids, means a superpower discovered by one bacterium can spread like wildfire through completely different bacterial species. Imagine one soldier figuring out how to disable a tank, then instantly sharing that knowledge electronically with the entire enemy army, regardless of their division. That's how devastatingly fast resistance genes, like the infamous blaNDM-1 that neutralizes some of our last-resort antibiotics, can sweep across the microbial world, turning treatable infections into deadly threats (and potentially hiking mortality rates by up to 40% for some infections, as the WHO warns).

Decoding the Enemy's Playbook and Mapping the Battlefield

So, how do we eavesdrop on these microscopic manoeuvres? We've developed two incredible intelligence tools:

Genetic Codebreaking (Genomics): Whole-genome sequencing (WGS) is our decoder ring. It lets us read the entire genetic instruction manual of a captured bacterial enemy. Instantly, we can see: What resistance weapons (genes) does it carry? Is it related to the bacteria infecting the patient next door (revealing transmission)? Did it just invent a new way to resist our drugs (a novel mutation)? WGS transforms bacteria from anonymous threats into known adversaries with identifiable fingerprints, turning outbreak investigations from slow-motion replays into live-action intelligence briefings. We're moving towards a future where sequencing results land on doctors' desks almost as fast as the initial lab report, guiding treatment in near real-time.

Situational Awareness (Ecology): Knowing the enemy's code isn't enough. We need to know where they are, how they're moving, and what conditions favour them. This is where ecological data comes in – it's our battlefield map. Are resistant strains hiding out on hospital bed rails, lurking in sink drains, or hitching rides between patients? Is heavy antibiotic use in one ward creating a perfect breeding ground? By overlaying this environmental and movement data onto our genomic intel, we get the full picture. Finding the same genetic fingerprint in multiple patients and on the sink they share? That's not a coincidence; it's a confirmed transmission route and a target for immediate action.

Real-Time Intel, Real-World Counterattacks

This fusion of codebreaking and battlefield mapping isn't just academic; it's triggering rapid, targeted counter-offensives:

Case File: The Klebsiella Containment: Imagine alarms flare – a patient's Klebsiella infection is resistant to our big-gun carbapenem antibiotics, thanks to the notorious blaNDM-1 gene. Instead of weeks of waiting, WGS screams confirmation within 48 hours. It reveals the gene is on an easily shared plasmid (high alert!) and matches isolates from two other patients. The genetic fingerprints are nearly identical – active transmission is happening now. Simultaneously, ecological scouts swab the environment, guided by patient locations. Bingo. The same strain is found chilling in a sink drain.

The Response: No more guesswork. A rapid response team deploys:

Containment: Affected patients are isolated, maybe with dedicated staff – building firewalls against further spread.

Targeted Sweeps: Knowing the exact strain allows rapid screening of other patients to find silent carriers before they spread it.

Precision Cleaning: Forget general scrubbing; that sink drain and surrounding areas get intense, targeted decontamination – neutralizing the identified reservoir.

Smarter Tactics: Doctors, armed with the resistance profile, immediately switch to effective alternative antibiotics, saving the patients and preserving carbapenems for future battles.

Case File: The MRSA Trail: A cluster of nasty MRSA skin infections pops up among high school athletes across town. Are they linked? WGS acts like a forensic genealogist. Sequencing the MRSA from each student reveals they're virtually identical – confirming a single outbreak strain is making the rounds, likely via shared gym equipment or locker rooms. Tiny variations in the genetic code can even sketch out a transmission tree – who likely got it from whom.

The Response: Public health officials don't have to rely solely on interviews. They can rapidly pinpoint hotspots, educate coaches and athletes on specific hygiene measures (like cleaning wrestling mats or not sharing towels), and ensure facilities are properly disinfected, potentially stopping the spread weeks faster than before.

Outsmarting Evolution Itself

By harnessing the power to watch microbial evolution in real-time, we're fundamentally changing the rules of engagement. We're shifting from being reactive historians of resistance to proactive defenders. We're turning mountains of complex genetic and ecological data into actionable intelligence, allowing us to intervene faster, smarter, and more precisely than ever before. This isn't just about fighting bacteria; it's about understanding and, hopefully, outsmarting evolution itself to keep our life-saving medicines working for generations to come. The invisible enemy is adapting, but now, we're finally watching – and learning how to fight back in real time.

Okay, let's step away from the microscope and look around. That tiny battle we've been watching in petri dishes? It's escaped. Antimicrobial Resistance (AMR) isn't just some sci-fi concept brewing in a lab anymore; it's out here, walking among us, woven into the very fabric of how we live, think, and connect.

Think of antibiotics as once-mighty superheroes. For decades, they saved us, miracle workers against invisible invaders. But we haven't treated them like the precious resource they are. Now, the villains – the bacteria and other microbes – are learning, adapting, shrugging off our best weapons. This isn't just a health headline; it's a looming shadow. The experts, like the WHO, aren't mincing words: if we don't change course, by 2050, these "superbugs" could claim 10 million lives every single year. That's more than cancer. Imagine a world where a simple infection, a scraped knee, or routine surgery becomes a life-or-death gamble again. That's the future AMR is writing, unless we grab the pen.

Why is this happening? It's easy to point fingers at complex biology, but the truth is messier, more human. It lives in the conversations we have, the beliefs we hold, the pressures we feel.

Remember that nagging cough? The one that just wouldn't quit? Many of us, somewhere deep down, have felt that urge: "Maybe an antibiotic will just knock this out." Even when we know it's likely a virus (which antibiotics can't touch), the hope for a quick fix is powerful. Surveys confirm this isn't just you or me; it's a global phenomenon

[Source: WHO Multi-Country Survey, 2015]. People mistakenly believe antibiotics are cure-alls for colds and flu. This belief fuels pressure on doctors, who are often caught between guidelines and a suffering patient desperate for relief [Source: Studies on patient-doctor interactions].

These aren't just simple mistakes. They're tangled up in culture. What does "getting better" mean in different communities? How much faith do we place in a pill versus letting our bodies heal? In some places, advertising shouts about miracle drugs. Elsewhere, taking time off work for a lingering virus just isn't an option, making a prescription feel like the only practical choice. Imagine digging into why some cultures might value certain types of medicine over others – it's a complex tapestry of tradition, trust, and lived experience that shapes whether someone demands, accepts, or refuses an antibiotic.

And just telling people "don't misuse antibiotics" often doesn't cut it. Think about it: Do you truly feel personally threatened by AMR right now? Does it seem like a distant, abstract problem? What's the immediate payoff for you to skip that antibiotic you think might help? Are doctors easy and affordable to see, or is it simpler to use leftover pills or get them from a less-than-official source? [Source: Health Belief Model; Theory of Planned Behavior]. These aren't just hypothetical questions; they reflect the real-world calculations people make every day. Convenience, cost, what friends and family do – it all plays a part. Shockingly, it's estimated that maybe half of all antibiotics used globally aren't needed or aren't taken correctly [Source: CDC estimates; WHO data].

So, if the problem breathes in our communities, the solutions must live there too. We need to move beyond just clinic walls and lab benches.

Picture this: In a village where the religious leader is the most trusted voice, imagine them weaving messages about responsible antibiotic use into their sermons. Not just as medical advice, but as an act of community care, of protecting future generations. This isn't just theory; groups working on the ground see how faith leaders can gently challenge myths and guide people toward better health choices, framing stewardship as a shared value [Source: Reports from NGOs engaging Faith-Based Organizations].

Or think about schools. Kids soak up knowledge like sponges. Programs like "e-Bug" in Europe show that teaching children about germs, hygiene, and how medicines work can plant seeds for a lifetime of smarter choices. These kids then go home and become little health ambassadors for their families [Source: e-Bug project].

And it doesn't stop with humans. The "One Health" idea reminds us we're connected – people, animals, the environment. Huge amounts of antibiotics are used in farming, sometimes just to make animals grow faster, not because they're sick [Source: FAO/OIE/WHO reports]. This breeds resistance that can jump to humans. Changing this means talking to farmers, understanding their economic realities, finding new ways to keep animals healthy, and maybe even creating demand for food raised without routine antibiotic use. It's about understanding the whole system, from farm to fork [Source: Research in agricultural economics].

Ultimately, seeing AMR as a social challenge means recognizing it's our challenge. It belongs to all of us – doctors, yes, but also sociologists, teachers, parents, community elders, farmers, politicians, you. We need to get creative, empathetic, and local. We need initiatives born from within communities, led by trusted voices, speaking languages people understand.

The fight against the superbugs won't be won solely with new drugs. It will be won in kitchens, classrooms, community halls, and fields. It will be won by changing habits, challenging assumptions, and recognizing that protecting these miracle medicines is a profound act of shared responsibility. It's time to bring the battle home.

Decoding Resistance at the Molecular Frontier

The Whispering Plague: How Tiny Renegades Arm Bacteria Against Us

Forget isolated germs. Picture the microscopic world as a bustling, clandestine city humming with constant chatter. Beneath the surface of our awareness, bacteria operate a vast, invisible intelligence network. And the hottest commodity traded in this hidden economy? The blueprints for shrugging off our life-saving antibiotics. This isn't slow-burn evolution; it's a high-speed, underground arms trade, fueled by microscopic couriers called mobile genetic elements. Think of them as genetic smugglers, primarily plasmids and transposons, passing secrets from microbe to microbe in a process called horizontal gene transfer (HGT).

This isn't just parent-to-child inheritance – that's the slow, steady way. HGT is like instant messaging for superpowers, allowing bacteria to gear up against our medicines almost overnight. It's why your doctor warns about finishing antibiotics, why infections we once dismissed are becoming deadly. This isn't some far-off sci-fi scenario; the World Health Organization calls antimicrobial resistance (AMR) a top global emergency, a silent pandemic already claiming millions of lives. If we don't change the game, projections warn of a future where 10 million people could die each year from untreatable infections by 2050 – that's more than cancer claims today. This unseen network is actively plotting our medical future.

Plasmids: The High-Speed Getaway Cars of Resistance

Imagine tiny, rogue circles of DNA floating inside bacteria, separate from the main genetic instruction manual. These are plasmids – think of them as compact, highly mobile USB drives packed with optional software, including potent defense codes against antibiotics. Their favourite trick for spreading these codes is conjugation, a process often dubbed "bacterial sex." It's less romantic, more like a microscopic back-alley deal: one bacterium extends a tiny, tube-like grappling hook (a pilus) to another and directly injects a copy of its plasmid. Suddenly, one resistant gangster can arm an entire neighbourhood of previously harmless bacteria.

Cutting-edge science is revealing just how slick this operation is. Some plasmids are like master keys, incredibly "promiscuous," able to sneak their genetic cargo into a wide variety of bacterial species. Others are more selective. Disturbingly, research shows that sometimes, the very presence of antibiotics – our intended weapon – can trigger more frantic plasmid swapping, like throwing gasoline on a fire we're trying to put out. Tracking notorious plasmids, like those carrying the infamous NDM-1 gene (which grants resistance to powerful carbapenem antibiotics), reveals how they've hitchhiked across the globe, hopping between different bacteria on super-successful plasmid "chassis" types. Understanding which plasmids are the major players and how they spread is like mapping a criminal underworld.

Transposons: The Shape-Shifting DNA Hitchhikers

Then there are the transposons, the "jumping genes." These aren't independent drifters like plasmids; they're segments of DNA that act like genetic acrobats, leaping from one spot in the bacterial genome to another. Think "cut and paste" or "copy and paste" on a molecular level.

Why should we care about these genetic gymnasts? Because they often carry resistance genes with them. A transposon armed with, say, tetracycline resistance can leap from a quiet spot on the bacterial chromosome onto one of those high-speed plasmids. Voila! That plasmid, already a potent delivery vehicle, now carries an extra weapon. When it gets transferred via conjugation, it delivers a multi-drug resistance package deal. It's how bacteria assemble devastating arsenals. We see this constantly in labs: complex structures called "integrons," which are like modular cargo bays for snapping up resistance genes, are frequently found embedded within transposons, which are themselves riding on plasmids. It's layers upon layers of mobility, creating super-resistant bugs.

Jamming the Network: A New Strategy Against the Invisible Enemy

If these mobile elements are the getaway cars and smugglers driving the resistance crisis, maybe we shouldn't just focus on neutralizing the weapons (the resistance mechanisms) or killing the individual bacteria. What if we could disrupt the smuggling network itself? What if we could block the transfer?

Targeting conjugation – stopping bacteria from passing those plasmid USB drives – is a radical, emerging idea. The potential beauty? It might put less direct life-or-death pressure on the bacteria compared to traditional antibiotics. If you're not trying to kill them outright, just stop them from sharing secrets, they might be slower to develop resistance to the blocker itself.

Consider the Common Misery: The UTI

Think about a urinary tract infection (UTI), often caused by E. coli. Inside the bladder, you might have a mix of bacteria – some susceptible to antibiotics, some already resistant thanks to plasmids. When you take an antibiotic, the resistant ones survive and, crucially, start rapidly sharing their resistance plasmids with the susceptible neighbours via conjugation. Soon, the whole bacterial population is armed, the antibiotic fails, and the infection rages on.

Now, imagine adding a conjugation inhibitor alongside the antibiotic. This molecule acts like a signal jammer, preventing the bacteria from forming that pilus bridge or transferring the plasmid DNA. The resistant bacteria are still there, but they can't share their cheat codes. The antibiotic can now effectively wipe out the still-susceptible majority, potentially clearing the infection. This strategy aims to contain resistance, preventing its wildfire spread during treatment. While dedicated drugs are still mostly experimental (though some existing meds show surprising side effects like blocking conjugation in labs), the principle is sound. It's about managing the microbial community and its lines of communication, not just waging total war.

The Takeaway

The antibiotic resistance crisis isn't just about stronger germs; it's about a hyper-efficient, hidden network facilitating their rise. Plasmids and transposons are the unsung architects of this threat, the couriers and shape-shifters dealing in survival codes. Understanding their shadowy operations is critical. And perhaps, by learning to jam their signals and disrupt their trade routes, we can find clever new ways to protect our medicines and ourselves from the whispering plague beneath the surface.

Beyond Germs: Meet the Slime Cities That Laugh Off Our Weapons

Forget lone-wolf bacteria floating aimlessly. Picture this: vast, invisible empires built beneath our notice, thriving in places we desperately need to be sterile. These aren't just random clumps of microbes; they're biofilms – bustling, organized communities, the bacterial equivalent of fortified cities, built from their own living slime.

This isn't your garden-variety pond scum. This is a meticulously engineered shield, a gooey fortress wall known scientifically as the Extracellular Polymeric Substance (EPS) matrix. Think of it as bacterial concrete, mixed from sugars, proteins, fats, and even DNA strands ripped from their fallen comrades. It's this living glue that turns a random gathering of bacteria into a near-impenetrable stronghold, shrugging off threats that would obliterate their free-floating cousins.

Why Your Antibiotics Bounce Right Off

These slime cities are masters of defense. First, there's the sheer physical barrier. Imagine trying to hose down a fortress built of sticky, dense jelly – the water (or antibiotic) just can't easily soak through to the inhabitants hiding deep inside. Researchers have seen antibiotic concentrations plummet dramatically within the biofilm's depths, often falling way below the knockout dose needed to actually harm the bacteria nestled within. It's like trying to put out a castle fire with a leaky garden hose.

But it's smarter than just a thick wall. This isn't passive goo; it's reactive armor. The components of the slime can actively grab onto invading antibiotic molecules, neutralizing them like microscopic anti-missile systems. They disarm the weapons before they even get close to the target bacteria. It's no wonder bacteria hunkered down in a biofilm can sometimes withstand antibiotic concentrations a thousand times higher than what would kill them out in the open.

Life in the Slow Lane: The Hidden Resistors

Inside these microbial fortresses, life is different. Deep within the slimy layers, oxygen and nutrients become scarce. It's like the packed inner districts of a city under siege. In response, many bacteria slow way down, entering a state of near-hibernation. These aren't just slowpokes; they're survivalists, often called "persister cells."

Here's the kicker: many of our best antibiotics are designed to attack bacteria when they're actively growing and dividing. But persister cells? They're essentially playing dead. They don't need to build cell walls or replicate DNA rapidly, so the antibiotics targeting those processes just wash right over them, ineffective. These hidden resistors are the reason biofilm infections – think stubborn chronic wounds, recurring lung infections in cystic fibrosis, or infected implants – are so maddeningly difficult to clear. They survive the antibiotic onslaught and, once the coast is clear, emerge to rebuild the city, leading to relapse. Some estimates suggest these slime cities are involved in a staggering 80% of chronic infections.

Whispers in the Slime: Sharing Survival Secrets

If that wasn't enough, these crowded cities are hotbeds for information sharing. Bacteria in close quarters constantly exchange genetic material – it's called horizontal gene transfer. Think of it like a spy network passing critical intel – in this case, blueprints for antibiotic resistance. A single bacterium that develops or acquires a new defense mechanism can quickly share that trait with its neighbors, rapidly upgrading the entire community's defenses.

Storming the Fortress: New Battle Plans

So, how do you fight an enemy that builds its own shields, plays dead, and shares secrets? The battle plan is shifting. Instead of just trying to poison individual soldiers, scientists are figuring out how to dismantle the fortress itself or disrupt its internal operations.

One strategy is to bring in the demolition crews: enzymes. Special enzymes can chew through the EPS matrix – dissolving the "concrete" – breaking down key components like DNA or specific sugars. Weakening the walls makes the inhabitants vulnerable, allowing antibiotics or even our own immune cells to finally get in and do their job.

Another clever tactic targets their communication network. Bacteria coordinate their actions, including biofilm building, using chemical signals – a process called quorum sensing. It's like their internet or radio system. By using "quorum sensing inhibitors" (QSIs), we can essentially jam their signals. Imagine blocking the command to "build walls!" or "release toxins!" This can prevent biofilms from forming properly, or even destabilize existing ones, making the bacteria confused, disorganized, and much easier targets for conventional treatments.

The Front Lines: Wounds and Implants

Think about a wound that just won't heal. Chances are, it's become a battlefield dominated by a biofilm. Standard antiseptics and antibiotics struggle against that slimy defense. But imagine applying a cream containing QSIs – molecules that silence the bacteria's chatter, preventing them from organizing their defenses, allowing the healing process to finally gain ground.

Or consider medical devices – catheters, artificial joints, heart valves. These sterile surfaces are prime real estate for biofilms. Once established, they can seed dangerous infections. Researchers are now designing materials coated with matrix-busting enzymes or signal-jamming QSIs, aiming to make these surfaces inhospitable fortresses from the start – booby-trapping them against microbial invaders.

The Takeaway

Biofilms aren't just clumps of germs; they are sophisticated, resilient microbial societies that have evolved incredible defenses. They challenge our traditional approaches to fighting infection. But by recognizing them as the organized communities they are, we're developing smarter weapons – ones that tear down their walls, scramble their communications, and disrupt their very way of life. The fight is far from over, but we're finally learning how to attack the fortress, not just the soldiers within.

The Bug's Secret Weapon: It's Not Just Armor, It's a Whole New Engine

We hear a lot about antibiotic resistance, this terrifying shadow looming over modern medicine [Source: WHO Report on AMR, 2024]. We often picture bacteria like tiny knights, building thicker walls or pumps to eject our drug "arrows" [Source: Nature Reviews Microbiology, 2022]. But the real story is getting wilder, more like a sci-fi thriller happening at a microscopic level.

Imagine this: you hit a bacterium with an antibiotic, trying to shut down one of its essential operations. Instead of just blocking the attack, the bug rewires its entire internal system. It's not just defending; it's fundamentally changing how it lives to survive the assault [Source: Cell Host & Microbe, 2023]. This isn't just defense; it's adaptation on the fly – a metabolic metamorphosis.

Masters of Improvisation: How Bugs Rewire to Resist

Think of a microbe's metabolism as its intricate network of power plants and factories – the chemical reactions making energy and building blocks [Source: Current Opinion in Microbiology, 2023]. When we attack one part of this network, resistant bugs become masters of improvisation:

Switching Fuel Lines: If an antibiotic blocks their favorite sugar-processing pathway, they might just reroute, tapping into a different energy source entirely, leaving the drug hitting a dead end [Source: mBio, 2022].

Running Damage Control: Some ramp up specific internal factories to churn out molecules that repair the damage caused by the drug, or even molecules that chemically neutralize the antibiotic itself [Source: PLOS Pathogens, 2023].

Going Low Power Mode: A really sneaky trick involves changes in their main energy circuits (like glycolysis and the TCA cycle) [Source: Frontiers in Microbiology, 2023]. Some bacteria can enter a state of near-dormancy, like putting their metabolism into low gear. Antibiotics that target active processes (like building cell walls or making proteins) just fly right past these "persister" cells [Source: Nature Communications, 2022]. These sleepy survivors are likely culprits behind those frustrating infections that keep coming back, hiding out until the antibiotic pressure is off [Source: FEMS Microbiology Reviews, 2023].

Sending Out Interference: Sometimes, the very byproducts of their new metabolic routes can mess with the antibiotic's function or trigger internal alarms that bolster the cell's defenses [Source: eLife, 2022].

The consequences aren't abstract; this metabolic adaptability is a key reason why infections that used to be treatable are becoming deadly, contributing to millions of deaths worldwide each year [Source: The Lancet, 2022].

Turning the Tables: Hitting Them Where They Live (Metabolically)

If bugs use their metabolism as a survival tool, what if we target that? It's like finding out the villain's secret power source and pulling the plug. This is the exciting idea behind metabolic inhibitors – drugs designed not necessarily to kill directly, but to sabotage the bug's internal machinery [Source: ACS Infectious Diseases, 2023; inspired by concepts potentially explored in future NEJM articles, e.g., NEJM 2025].

The goal is to find metabolic choke points – essential processes for the pathogen, especially when it's under attack or causing infection – that are different or less important in our own human cells [Source: Trends in Pharmacological Sciences, 2022]. Think of unique bacterial pathways for making fats (like FASII) or certain amino acids [Source: Journal of Medicinal Chemistry, 2023]. Researchers are hunting for molecules that can precisely jam these microbial gears, weakening the pathogen or, crucially, making it vulnerable again to our existing antibiotics [Source: Drug Resistance Updates, 2022].

The One-Two Punch: The Real Magic of Combination Therapy

Here's where it gets really promising: teaming up. Imagine hitting the bug with a standard antibiotic and a metabolic inhibitor simultaneously [Source: Nature Reviews Drug Discovery, 2021]. This tag-team approach is powerful:

Lowering the Defenses: Crippling the bug's metabolism can often make it susceptible again to an antibiotic it had previously shrugged off [Source: Science Translational Medicine, 2020].

Harder to Resist: It's much tougher for a bug to simultaneously develop workarounds for two completely different types of attacks [Source: Cell Chemical Biology, 2022]. It's like trying to dodge punches coming from two directions at once.

Bringing Old Weapons Back: The MRSA Story

Let's look at MRSA (Methicillin-resistant Staphylococcus aureus), the infamous superbug plaguing hospitals and communities [Source: Clinical Infectious Diseases, 2023]. We know MRSA employs specific metabolic tricks to fuel its resistance and virulence [Source: Journal of Bacteriology, 2022].

Now, researchers are showing that if you block certain metabolic pathways in MRSA – say, key steps in making the amino acid arginine – you can dramatically weaken its resistance to methicillin-type antibiotics (like oxacillin) [Source: Antimicrobial Agents and Chemotherapy, 2023; mSphere, 2021]. Imagine needing 64 times less oxacillin to kill the bug just by adding a metabolic blocker [Illustrative Example]. Suddenly, an old, seemingly useless antibiotic might be back in the fight, thanks to this metabolic sabotage. This isn't just theory; compounds targeting

MRSA's metabolism are showing real promise in lab and animal studies.

Beyond MRSA: A Widespread Strategy

This isn't just an S. aureus trick. The same logic applies to other nightmare bugs:

Mycobacterium tuberculosis (TB): Known for hiding out metabolically. Targeting its unique energy pathways (like how it eats cholesterol) could finally shorten the brutally long TB treatment [Source: Nature Reviews Microbiology, 2021; Trends in Microbiology, 2023].

Pseudomonas aeruginosa: Forms tough, slimy biofilms. Understanding and disrupting the unique metabolism within these biofilms could break them up and let antibiotics in [Source: NPJ Biofilms and Microbiomes, 2022].

Acinetobacter baumannii: A master of survival in hospitals. Finding its essential metabolic weak spots is key to fighting this multi-drug resistant threat [Source: Gut Microbes, 2023].

While we're still waiting for these combination therapies to become mainstream clinical practice, the pipeline is buzzing with activity [Source: Expert Opinion on Drug Discovery, 2023]. The big hurdles are crafting inhibitors that are laser-focused on microbes, pack a punch, and are safe and effective in humans.

Conclusion: A New Front in the Superbug War

Understanding how bugs rewire themselves isn't just fascinating science – it's cracking open a new front in the war against resistance. By looking beyond simple shields and targeting the very life processes of these pathogens, especially their metabolic flexibility, we're finding their hidden vulnerabilities. Sabotaging their metabolism, particularly alongside our existing antibiotics, feels less like just fighting back and more like outsmarting the enemy. It's a complex battleground, but one where innovative science offers a powerful, perhaps revolutionary, path forward to reclaim ground against the infections that threaten us most. We're learning to fight smarter, not just harder.

The Ghost in the Machine: How Bacteria Use Epigenetic Tricks to Defy Our Drugs

Imagine the fight against antibiotic-resistant bacteria. We often picture it like trench warfare: bacteria dig in, developing tough genetic mutations like shields and armor over long, grueling battles. But what if there's more to it? What if bacteria have a secret weapon, a kind of battlefield improvisation, allowing them to change tactics on the fly without rewriting their fundamental genetic orders?

Welcome to the shadowy world of bacterial epigenetics – think of it as the software running on the bacteria's genetic hardware. It's about changes in how genes behave, not changes in the genes themselves. Like adding sticky notes or highlights to their DNA instruction manual, bacteria can quickly tweak which commands get read loudly, whispered, or ignored entirely. This isn't about slow evolution; it's about rapid adaptation, a nimble dance of survival.

The main trick in their epigenetic playbook is DNA methylation. Tiny chemical tags, like molecular Post-it notes, get slapped onto the DNA by specialized enzymes (think of them as microscopic scribes called MTases). These tags don't alter the DNA's core text, but they can act like dimmer switches or volume controls for nearby genes. Need to pump out that incoming antibiotic? An epigenetic tweak might crank up the volume on the gene controlling the cellular pump, kicking the drug out before it does harm. Facing a different stress? Another tweak might silence a gene to conserve energy or change the bacterium's outer coat to hide from immune cells.

This isn't some niche strategy; it's practically universal. It turns out over 90% of bacteria we've looked at have these MTase scribes, constantly annotating their genetic blueprints. It's like discovering that almost every soldier carries not just a rifle, but also a kit for camouflage and quick-change disguises. This epigenetic flexibility allows bacteria to flip genes on or off with startling speed – controlling everything from their attack strategies (virulence) and ability to form protective slime cities (biofilms) to, crucially, their resistance to our best medicines. It's a system that lets them respond to threats now, rather than waiting generations for a lucky genetic mutation to arise.

Here's where it gets exciting for us: if bacteria are using this epigenetic code to resist our drugs, what if we could hack it? What if we could develop "eraser" molecules that wipe away those resistance-boosting sticky notes? Or "blockers" that stop the MTase scribes from writing them in the first place? This is the dawn of bacterial epigenetic therapy.

The idea is tantalizing: by interfering with these epigenetic controls, we might disarm bacteria, making them vulnerable to antibiotics they previously laughed off. This approach holds particular promise against "persister" cells – the stubborn bacteria that go dormant during treatment, hiding out like sleeper agents, only to reawaken later and cause infection relapse. Epigenetics seems to be key in controlling this dangerous hide-and-seek behavior. Targeting these controls could potentially prevent bacteria from hiding or flush them out, making them susceptible again.

Consider the notorious superbug, Pseudomonas aeruginosa. This villain is a master of resistance, causing persistent, hard-to-treat infections, especially in hospitals and for people with conditions like cystic fibrosis. We're learning that Pseudomonas heavily relies on its complex epigenetic system. Its MTase scribes are busy regulating its weapons, its biofilm fortresses, and its drug defenses. Early lab experiments are showing real promise: using prototype "epi-inhibitor" drugs can sometimes slash the amount of antibiotic needed to kill Pseudomonas, effectively reviving old drugs. These inhibitors can also sabotage biofilm formation, breaking down the bacteria's protective communities.

Of course, it's not simple. We need tools precise enough to target the bacterial scribes without messing with our own human cellular machinery (we use epigenetics too!). And delivering these tools deep into infection sites, especially slimy biofilms, is a challenge.

But the path is illuminated. We're realizing that the genetic code is only part of the story. Bacteria are dynamic, adaptable foes using layers of regulation we're just beginning to understand. By deciphering and learning to manipulate their epigenetic "software," we might just find the counter-hacks we desperately need. The fight against antibiotic resistance isn't just about breaking down walls; it's also about rewriting the enemy's hidden instructions. The future of tackling these persistent infections might lie in silencing the whispers of the ghost in the bacterial machine.

The Fungal Frontier: Confronting Antifungal Resistance

The Unseen Siege: How Fungi Fight Back Against Our Medicines

Imagine trying to defeat an enemy that doesn't just resist, but actively outsmarts your attacks. That's the battle we face against pathogenic fungi. These aren't simple organisms; they're microscopic survivors armed with sophisticated defenses, turning our life-saving antifungal drugs into mere annoyances. Think of it less like medicine and more like laying siege to a cleverly defended fortress, one that learns and adapts. Let's peek inside their armory and uncover their three favorite battle plans:

1. The Pump-and-Dump Defense: Cellular Eviction Squads

Picture tiny, tireless bouncers stationed at every entrance of the fungal cell. These aren't just passive guards; they're hyper-efficient efflux pumps, protein machines embedded in the cell's border wall. Their mission? Grab any unwelcome intruders – like our antifungal drugs – and forcefully eject them before they can cause trouble inside. Fungi have whole families of these pumps (like the ABC and MFS crews), ready to be activated.

It gets smarter. Fungi facing attack can actually build more pumps, turning a trickle of defense into a flood. Genes like CDR1, CDR2, and MDR1 in notorious fungi like Candida species are the blueprints for these pumps. When the fungus overexpresses these genes (think: putting the pump factories into overdrive), especially against common drugs like fluconazole, it becomes incredibly difficult to treat. Sometimes, rogue 'commanders' within the cell (mutated transcription factors like Tac1p or Mrr1p) order these pumps to run constantly, making the fungus born resistant, ready for a fight even before the first drug dose hits. This isn't just theory; scientists can directly measure the increased pump activity in drug-resistant strains, proving these cellular bouncers are major players on the microbial battlefield.

2. The Master of Disguise: Altering the Bullseye

Our antifungal drugs are often like highly specific keys, designed to fit perfectly into a vital lock (a specific enzyme or protein) within the fungal cell, gumming up the works. Azole drugs, for instance, target the machinery (ERG11 gene product) that builds the fungal cell's unique wall component, ergosterol. Echinocandins go after the enzyme (FKS gene product) responsible for weaving the structural backbone of the cell wall.

But what if the fungus could subtly change the shape of the lock? That's exactly what happens with target site mutations. A tiny tweak, just a single amino acid change in the drug's target protein, can be like filing down a key groove or changing the tumblers. The drug-key no longer fits snugly, its binding power plummets, and it becomes useless. We see this play out tragically in the real world. Certain mutations in the FKS genes are notorious for causing resistance to echinocandins in dangerous species like Candida glabrata and the menacing Candida auris. Similarly, the widespread ERG11 mutation (TR34/L98H) in Aspergillus fumigatus, sometimes linked to fungicide use in agriculture, makes this common mold resistant to azoles, directly impacting patients across continents. Detecting these specific "disguises" is now a key part of diagnosing resistant infections.

3. The Survivalist's Playbook: Weathering the Storm

Sometimes, it's not about directly blocking or ejecting the drug, but simply surviving the initial onslaught. When fungi sense the stress of an antifungal attack, they trigger complex stress response pathways – activating their internal 'emergency services'. While this might not grant them superhero-level resistance immediately, it buys them precious time, allowing them to endure the drug long enough for more permanent defenses (like those pump upgrades or target disguises) to emerge.

Key operatives in this survival game include proteins like Hsp90. Think of Hsp90 as a molecular chaperone, a cellular mechanic that rushes around stabilizing other proteins, including slightly damaged drug targets or newly built efflux pumps, helping them function even under duress or with minor mutations. Blocking Hsp90 can actually make resistant fungi vulnerable again! Another critical player is the calcineurin pathway, essential for patching up the cell wall and managing membrane damage caused by drugs. Shutting down this pathway also makes fungi more susceptible. It's clear that bolstering their general resilience is a core fungal tactic – hunkering down to survive the siege.

From the Lab Bench to the Bedside: Why This Matters

Understanding these fungal countermeasures isn't just fascinating science; it's life-saving intelligence for doctors on the front lines:

Smarter Treatments: Knowing how a fungus is resisting helps choose the right weapon. If a Candida infection is resistant due to overactive pumps but the drug target itself is fine, switching to a drug class that ignores the pumps (like an echinocandin) might work. But if an FKS mutation is detected, echinocandins are off the table, and doctors need alternatives like amphotericin B or different strategies. Modern labs are increasingly using molecular "reconnaissance" to spot these resistance mechanisms.

Case File: The Resistant Mold (Aspergillus fumigatus): A patient is struggling with an invasive Aspergillus infection. The go-to azole drug isn't working. Tests reveal the infamous TR34/L98H mutation. This tells the doctor that simply upping the azole dose is futile. The battle plan shifts: perhaps bringing in the heavy artillery (liposomal amphotericin B) or employing a two-pronged attack (combination therapy, maybe pairing an azole with an echinocandin) to hit the fungus from multiple angles, bypassing its primary defense.

Case File: The Global Threat (Candida auris): This formidable yeast is like a master strategist, often equipped with multiple resistance mechanisms simultaneously – super-charged pumps, altered targets for several drug types, and robust stress defenses. Treating a C. auris infection is a complex challenge, requiring extensive testing to probe its specific weaknesses and often demanding newer drugs or combination therapies tailored to the individual strain. Its ability to deploy a full arsenal of resistance tactics explains its frightening mortality rates in vulnerable patients.

The Ongoing Arms Race

Pathogenic fungi are not passive targets. They are dynamic, adaptable opponents employing an impressive array of defenses: tireless efflux pumps, shape-shifting target sites, and powerful survival protocols. As we learn more about their intricate strategies, we get better at diagnosing infections, choosing effective treatments, and critically, designing the next generation of antifungal weapons needed to breach these formidable fungal fortresses and win the fight against resistant infections.

The Whisper in the Fields, The Roar in the Clinic: How Farming Choices Echo in Our Fight Against Fungi

Imagine walking through a field, the air thick with the scent of earth and growing things. We see sprays protecting crops, ensuring the bounty reaches our tables. It seems like a world away from the sterile quiet of a hospital room where someone fights for breath against a relentless lung infection. But startling connections are emerging, like invisible threads linking the farmer's field to the patient's bedside. The chemicals we use to guard our harvests might be inadvertently training the very fungi that later threaten our most vulnerable.

The Double-Edged Sword: Our Shared Weapon Against Fungi

At the heart of this story is a class of chemicals called azoles. Think of them as a highly specialized key. In agriculture, they unlock protection for crops like cereals, fruits, and flowers against devastating fungal diseases. In medicine, a closely related set of azole keys (like itraconazole and voriconazole) are our frontline defense against dangerous fungal invaders in humans, particularly the notorious Aspergillus fumigatus that can haunt the lungs of those with weakened immunity.

Here's the dangerous twist: both the farmer's fungicide and the doctor's medicine target the exact same vulnerability in the fungus – its ability to build its protective cell wall. It's like having two armies using the same secret weapon against a common enemy. When azoles blanket our fields, gardens, and even treated wood, they kill off the susceptible fungi. But nature always finds a way. Fungi with tiny, random mutations that happen to resist the azoles survive. They thrive in the absence of competition, multiply, and spread their resilient offspring far and wide.

The environment becomes a vast, accidental training ground, breeding tougher fungal strains.

Aspergillus fumigatus: The Unseen Hitchhiker Turned Deadly Threat

We breathe in Aspergillus fumigatus spores constantly; they're part of the natural world, riding the breeze from soil and decaying leaves. For most of us, our immune system simply clears them out. But for someone recovering from a transplant, undergoing chemotherapy, or battling a chronic lung condition, inhaling these spores can be like inviting a Trojan horse. If the inhaled spore happens to be one of the "trained," azole-resistant strains emerging from the environment, the doctor's go-to medicines may suddenly fail.

The evidence is mounting, like ecological detective work. Scientists are finding resistant Aspergillus strains in patients that carry the exact same genetic resistance markers (like the infamous TR34/L98H) found in samples from agricultural soil, compost heaps, and even flower beds. Studies, particularly in places like the Netherlands with its vast flower bulb industry, have sounded the alarm, showing worryingly high levels (sometimes 10-20%) of azole-resistant Aspergillus in the environment – rates that mirror or even surpass those seen in hospitals. It paints a stark picture: a patient who has never personally received an azole drug can become infected with a resistant strain acquired directly from the air they breathe, its resistance forged in the fields outside.

Cultivating Resistance: How Farming Practices Turn Up the Volume

It's not just that we use fungicides, but how. Imagine the impact of:

Relentless Spraying: Repeated, season-long applications keep the pressure on, constantly selecting for the toughest fungi.

Waste Hotspots: Piles of azole-treated plant waste (like discarded bulbs or compost) can become five-star hotels for resistant fungi, allowing them to multiply exponentially and release clouds of resilient spores.

Monoculture Vulnerability: Vast fields of the same crop, often relying heavily on one type of fungicide, can create a perfect storm for resistance compared to more diverse farming systems.

Turning the Tide: From Recognition to Response

Understanding this environmental echo chamber isn't just academic; it demands action:

Rethinking Regulations: Health organizations and regulators worldwide are grappling with this, debating whether certain agricultural azoles, too similar to critical medicines, should be restricted or even banned to preserve our medical arsenal. The EU, for instance, explicitly weighs this environmental resistance risk when approving farm chemicals – a true "One Health" approach acknowledging that spraying a field can directly impact hospital outcomes.

Smarter Farming (Stewardship): This is about finesse, not just force. Using fungicides only when truly needed, rotating different types of chemicals so fungi don't adapt to just one, and embracing non-chemical methods (like hardier crop varieties or beneficial microbes) are crucial parts of Integrated Pest Management (IPM). Think of it as outsmarting the fungi rather than just trying to obliterate them. In the Netherlands, faced with the bulb waste issue, efforts began to find safer disposal methods and alternatives, trying to quiet the resistance incubator.

Environmental Watchdogs: Setting up surveillance systems to test air, soil, and water near farms for resistant fungi acts like an early warning system, helping us spot trouble brewing before it overwhelms clinics.

A Quick Note on Vineyards and Yeast: While azoles are used on grapevines, the strong, well-documented link between agricultural use and drug-resistant clinical infections points most powerfully to Aspergillus. Resistant Candida yeasts (like the alarming C. auris) are often more tied to healthcare settings. However, the underlying principle holds true: reducing the overall chemical pressure on fungi in any environment is a wise precaution against unexpected resistance popping up elsewhere.

Our Shared Breath, Our Shared Responsibility

The story of azole resistance is a powerful, unsettling reminder that human health, animal health, and the health of our environment are deeply intertwined. The quest to protect our food supply has cast an environmental shadow, potentially weakening our ability to heal the sick. Tackling this requires a united front – farmers using chemicals judiciously, scientists tracking the spread, regulators making tough choices, and doctors needing effective tools. We must listen to the environmental echo and act collaboratively, ensuring the whispers of resistance in the fields don't become an untreatable roar in our hospitals. Protecting our antifungal medicines for tomorrow means rethinking our actions in the environment today.

Decoding the Invisible Enemy: How Split-Second Science is Outsmarting Deadly Fungi

Imagine an enemy you can't see, one that learns, adapts, and turns medicine's trusted weapons useless. This isn't science fiction; it's the chilling reality of antifungal resistance. Fungi, often dismissed as simple organisms, are evolving defenses against our limited treatments at an alarming pace. What used to be manageable infections are morphing into life-or-death battles, especially for those with weakened immune systems where these invaders can claim lives with terrifying speed – sometimes over 50% don't survive, even with treatment.

For too long, we've been fighting this war with outdated intelligence. Traditional methods – growing fungi in a lab – are like waiting for smoke signals in an age of instant communication. Days, even weeks, can crawl by while doctors are forced to guess, choosing broad-spectrum treatments that might be like firing blanks at a resistant strain, or worse, causing unnecessary harm to the patient. All the while, the clock is ticking, and this blindfolded approach fuels the very resistance we're trying to combat. It's a desperate holding pattern when what we need is decisive action.

But science fights back. We're now deploying the biological equivalent of high-speed reconnaissance and code-breaking, tools that give us the upper hand in hours, not weeks. Forget waiting for the enemy to reveal itself slowly in a petri dish. Molecular diagnostics like quantitative PCR (qPCR) and next-generation sequencing (NGS) dive straight into the patient's sample – blood, fluid, tissue – and pull out the enemy's genetic blueprint.

qPCR: The Sharpshooter's Scope

Think of qPCR as a highly trained sniper. It's designed to zero in on specific, known targets. Does the patient have Candida albicans? Does it carry the notorious ERG11 mutation that laughs off fluconazole? qPCR can give a "yes" or "no" with astonishing speed, often within 2-4 hours. It's like instantly identifying the enemy's flag and knowing their primary weapon, allowing doctors to choose the right countermeasure immediately, potentially shaving critical days off the wait for lab-grown results.

NGS: The Full Intelligence Dossier

NGS, on the other hand, is like deploying a fleet of reconnaissance drones that map the entire battlefield. It doesn't just look for one or two known suspects; it sequences huge swathes of fungal DNA, revealing everything that's there. Is it a common foe, or something rare and unexpected? Are there multiple invaders working together? Crucially, NGS can uncover the enemy's entire playbook of resistance tricks – spotting not just known mutations across many genes, but potentially brand-new ones we haven't even seen before. This is vital as fungi constantly devise new ways to survive our drugs.

From Lab Bench to Bedside: Real-Time Victories

Let's see how this plays out:

Scenario 1: The Closing Window: A leukemia patient, vulnerable from chemo, develops severe pneumonia. The usual suspect is Aspergillus fumigatus, but is it the kind that shrugs off standard azole drugs? While the traditional culture lab begins its slow work, a qPCR test on lung fluid comes back in three hours. It screams positive for Aspergillus DNA and the TR34/L98H mutation – a known signal for azole resistance. Instead of gambling on a likely ineffective drug (voriconazole), the team immediately pivots to a different weapon, perhaps amphotericin B. They've bypassed days of potentially fatal delay, acting decisively based on rapid intelligence.

Scenario 2: The ICU Ghost: An ICU faces a mysterious cluster of hard-to-treat yeast infections. Standard tests are confused. NGS is deployed. Within a day, it unmasks the culprit: Candida auris, the notorious, often multidrug-resistant superbug known for haunting hospitals. But NGS does more – it reveals the specific genetic markers conferring resistance to multiple drug classes. This intel instantly guides doctors to the few remaining effective treatments (like amphotericin B) and triggers urgent infection control protocols to stop the ghost in its tracks.

The Future is Fast

Embracing qPCR and NGS isn't just about getting faster results; it's about fundamentally changing our strategy against fungal infections. It's about shifting from reactive guesswork to proactive, targeted strikes. It means giving patients the right drug, right away, dramatically improving their odds in a fight where every hour counts. It's also about being smarter stewards of the few antifungal drugs we have left, using them precisely to slow the tide of resistance.

Yes, there are hurdles – cost, making sure tests are reliable everywhere, teaching everyone how to read the complex intel NGS provides. But the need is undeniable. In the race against resistance, speed isn't just an advantage; it's survival. These rapid diagnostic tools are our indispensable allies, giving us the critical edge to protect patients and push back against the growing fungal threat.

Beyond the Mold: Reinventing Our Defense Against Fungal Invaders

Think of fungal infections less like a common cold and more like a shadowy siege. These microscopic invaders are increasingly outsmarting our defenses, especially for people whose bodies are already fighting other battles – like cancer patients or transplant recipients. The alarming truth is, our go-to antifungal weapons are getting old, and the fungi are learning how to shrug them off [Source: Fisher MC et al., Science, 2022]. We're facing growing resistance, nasty side effects, and drugs that just don't work on every type of fungal foe [Source: Perfect JR, Cold Spring Harb Perspect Med, 2017]. This isn't just a scientific problem; it's a human one, demanding fresh thinking and a dramatically expanded arsenal. We need new strategies – not just slightly better versions of the old ones, but entirely new ways to fight back, including turning the body's own defenses into fungal hunters and exploring the forgotten wisdom in nature's medicine cabinet.

1. Forging New Weapons: Outsmarting Fungi with Novel Drugs

For a while, the pipeline for new antifungals looked depressingly dry. But now, there's a buzz of activity. Scientists are crafting innovative molecules designed to hit fungi where it hurts – in ways our current drugs can't.

Shaking the Foundations (Targeting the Cell Wall):

Fosmanogepix: Imagine a construction crew building a faulty wall. That's what Fosmanogepix does. It messes with a crucial enzyme (Gwt1) that anchors vital proteins into the fungal cell wall, essentially making the fungus structurally unsound and less dangerous [Source: Pfaller MA et al., Antimicrob Agents Chemother, 2019]. It's showing promise against tough customers like Candida (even resistant ones), Aspergillus, and rare but deadly molds like Scedosporium [Source: Pappas PG et al., Open Forum Infect Dis, 2021]. Keep an eye out for major clinical trial results – the hope is it will prove highly effective, potentially turning the tide in infections that currently have grim outlooks [Source: ClinicalTrials.gov: NCT04240886 - evolving data].

Ibrexafungerp: This clever drug also targets the cell wall's building blocks (glucan synthase) but uses a different 'key' than existing drugs (echinocandins). This means it can sometimes work even when fungi have learned to resist the old keys [Source: Jallow S et al., Drugs, 2021]. Plus, it comes as a pill, a huge win for patients who might otherwise need IV drips. Already approved for vaginal yeast infections, its potential against invasive, body-wide infections is under intense investigation [Source: Spec A et al., Clin Infect Dis, 2023].

Stopping the Presses (Targeting Protein Production):

Olorofim: This drug is like a sniper hitting a single, vital target. It belongs to a whole new class (orotomides) and shuts down a fungal enzyme (DHODH) needed to make pyrimidines, essential building blocks for the fungus [Source: Oliver JD et al., PNAS, 2016]. Its superpower lies in its effectiveness against molds that laugh off other treatments, like drug-resistant Aspergillus and the notoriously difficult Lomentospora prolificans [Source: Hoenigl M et al., Lancet Microbe, 2021]. Late-stage trials will tell us exactly where this targeted weapon fits best in our clinical toolkit [Source: ClinicalTrials.gov: NCT03583164].

Teaching an Old Dog New Tricks (Improving Existing Classes):

Rezafungin: While it belongs to the established echinocandin family (targeting the cell wall), Rezafungin is the reimagined, high-performance version. Its standout feature? You only need it once a week [Source: Thompson

GR III et al., Lancet, 2023]. Compare that to the daily infusions of its older cousins! It's proven itself just as good as a standard daily drug for serious Candida infections [Source: Thompson GR III et al., Lancet, 2023]. This convenience isn't just nice; it could mean less time hooked up to an IV, potentially even finishing treatment at home – a game-changer for patient quality of life.

2. Rallying the Body's Own Defenses: Host-Directed Therapies (HDTs)

What if, instead of just poisoning the fungus, we could supercharge the patient's own immune system to fight it off? That's the revolutionary idea behind HDTs [Source: Cunha C et al., Front Immunol, 2018]. This approach is especially exciting for immunocompromised patients whose natural defenses are weakened. Think of it like:

Waking up Tired Immune Cells: Using drugs (like checkpoint inhibitors, famous in cancer therapy) to reignite immune cells that might have become exhausted during a long fungal fight [Source: Wójtowicz A et al., Cells, 2020].

Calling in Reinforcements: Administering natural body signals (like GM-CSF) to boost the number and power of fungus-fighting white blood cells [Source: Perfect JR, Cold Spring Harb Perspect Med, 2017].

Cutting Off Enemy Supply Lines: Modifying the body's own processes (like inflammation or iron availability) that fungi hijack to survive and thrive [Source: Akoumianaki T et al., Cell Host Microbe, 2016]. HDTs offer a tantalizing prospect: potentially working alongside traditional antifungals and being harder for fungi to develop resistance against. The challenge is mastering the complex interplay between our bodies and these invaders [Source: Richardson JP et al., Nat Rev Drug Discov, 2018].

3. Nature's Pharmacy: Unlocking Ancient Antifungal Secrets

Let's not forget the planet's own R&D department – nature! Plants, microbes, and essential oils are treasure troves of compounds with fungus-fighting potential.

Herbal Warriors & Aromatic Allies: Compounds from everyday sources like tea tree oil, garlic's allicin, and countless traditional medicinal plants show real promise in lab tests against Candida and other fungi [Source: Nazzaro F et al., Pharmaceuticals (Basel), 2017]. Ongoing research delves into how they work – do they poke holes in fungal membranes or shut down their enzymes? [Sources: e.g., Suleiman M et al., BMC Complement Med Ther, 2020]. The big hurdles are turning these natural wonders into reliable medicines: ensuring every batch is equally potent, proving they work inside the body (not just in a dish), and making sure they reach the infection site effectively [Source: Soliman SSM et al., Molecules, 2021]. Excitingly, some natural compounds seem to boost the power of conventional drugs, potentially allowing us to use lower doses and fight resistance through teamwork [Source: Doke SK et al., Front Microbiol, 2021].

4. From Brilliant Idea to Lifesaving Reality: The Path to Patients

Discovering a potential new antifungal is just the first step on a long, challenging road. To make a real difference, these innovations need to navigate:

The Trial Gauntlet: Rigorous testing in humans to prove they are safe and actually work better than, or add value to, what we already have.

The Approval Maze: Getting the green light from health authorities like the FDA and EMA.

The Doctor's Handbook: Being written into official treatment guidelines so doctors know when and how to use them.

Smarter Diagnosis: Pairing these new tools with faster, more accurate tests to identify the specific fungal enemy quickly.

Wise Use (Stewardship): Using these precious new drugs carefully to prevent resistance from emerging all over again.

Imagine This Scenario (Bringing it Home):

Picture Mr. Jones, 65, fighting leukemia. Chemotherapy has wiped out his immune cells, and now he has a fever. A dangerous yeast, Candida glabrata (often resistant to common drugs), is found in his blood. His kidneys aren't great, making one powerful option risky. But wait – Rezafungin, the once-weekly echinocandin, is known to work against this yeast [Source: Ham YY et al., J Antimicrob Chemother, 2021]. The doctor chooses Rezafungin. Mr. Jones gets his infusion, and because it's weekly, he might be able to leave the hospital sooner, managing his treatment without daily IV lines. That's not just good medicine; it's better living during a tough time.

Conclusion: A United Front Against a Rising Threat

The battle against fungal infections requires more than just wishful thinking; it demands relentless innovation. Groundbreaking drugs targeting new fungal weaknesses, clever strategies to empower our own immune systems, and the untapped potential of nature's remedies all offer vital streams of hope. But discovery alone isn't enough. We need dedication to push these advances through testing, approvals, and into smart, real-world practice. By embracing this multi-pronged attack – combining scientific brilliance with practical wisdom – we can forge a stronger shield against invasive fungal diseases and offer a brighter, healthier future for vulnerable patients everywhere.

Beyond Bacteria: Resistance in Viruses and Parasites

The Ghost in the Machine: Our High-Stakes Dance with Viral Shapeshifters

Forget battlefields of mud and metal. The most relentless war of our time is happening on a stage invisible to the naked eye, deep within the intricate machinery of our own cells. Our adversaries? Viruses – tiny, ingenious hijackers that have mastered the art of survival. And just when we think we have the upper hand, crafting clever drugs to block their path, they pull their oldest trick: they change. This isn't just evolution; it's a desperate, high-speed escape act we call antiviral resistance, and it's threatening to unravel our defenses against threats like the flu, COVID-19, and HIV. Staying ahead isn't just smart science; it's a race for our future health.

Imagine a virus, particularly one built from RNA like Influenza or SARS-CoV-2, as a frantic, slightly careless scribe. As it madly copies its genetic script to multiply, mistakes inevitably creep in – mutations. Think of them as typos in the viral code. Most are gibberish, weakening the virus. But every so often, a typo accidentally rewrites a crucial passage – maybe the exact spot where our antiviral drug is meant to latch on and disable it. Now, picture someone taking that drug. The medicine efficiently wipes out the original viruses, the ones it recognizes. But that one virus with the lucky typo? It slips through the net. With no competition, it flourishes, a lone survivor suddenly inheriting the kingdom within the patient. It's Darwinian evolution played out in biological hyperspeed, a ghost in the machine learning to dodge our bullets.

Flu: The Familiar Foe That Keeps Learning New Steps

Influenza is the seasoned veteran of this dance. It's constantly shuffling its genetic cards, forcing us to create new vaccines year after year. Our antiviral medicines, like oseltamivir (Tamiflu), target specific parts of the flu virus, like the neuraminidase enzyme it needs to escape infected cells. But the flu is a quick study. Specific typos, like the notorious H275Y mutation, can subtly alter that enzyme, making Tamiflu's grip less secure. Imagine researchers finding (as a hypothetical 2024 study might) that in some communities, 10-15% of tested H1N1 flu strains now shrugged off Tamiflu, all thanks to that specific genetic tweak. Suddenly, our go-to defense feels less certain.

How do we counter? We learn to dance too. Doctors and public health officials become strategists, monitoring which viral strains are circulating and which genetic "dodges" they possess. If tests show a patient has a Tamiflu-resistant flu, or if surveillance reveals widespread resistance in an outbreak, the playbook changes. Perhaps zanamivir (Relenza), another antiviral that often still works against these resistant strains, is moved to the front line. It's about being adaptable, keeping the virus guessing by switching partners on the dance floor, ensuring our limited moves remain effective.

COVID-19: A New Challenger Tests Our Latest Moves

The arrival of COVID-19 spurred an unprecedented scientific sprint, yielding antivirals like remdesivir and Paxlovid in record time. Remdesivir, for instance, cleverly sabotages the virus's copying machine, the RdRp enzyme. Yet, the ghost of resistance haunted even these new innovations. Whispers turned into reports, especially from patients with weakened immune systems fighting the virus for extended periods. In these prolonged internal battles, SARS-CoV-2 had more time, more chances to stumble upon those escape mutations.

Picture a (hypothetical) groundbreaking 2025 report chronicling this. Scientists might sequence virus samples from dozens of long-haul patients treated with remdesivir, identifying specific genetic typos in the RdRp gene that made the drug less potent. They might even quantify it: certain mutation patterns making the virus ten times less sensitive in the lab, tragically correlating with patients faring worse. It's a stark, urgent reminder: even our newest shields aren't impenetrable. This drives us to think smarter, perhaps deploying combinations of drugs right away for the most vulnerable, building higher walls against potential escape.

HIV: Hard-Won Wisdom from a Long Campaign

HIV, perhaps more than any other virus, has been our toughest teacher in this long war. Its astonishingly high mutation rate meant that early attempts to fight it with single drugs were disastrously short-lived. The virus simply learned to sidestep them too quickly. The revolution came with a radical idea: don't just block one door, barricade all the exits at once. This strategy, combination antiretroviral therapy (cART), uses three or more drugs simultaneously, each targeting a different critical step in HIV's lifecycle.

Think of it: the virus now needs to find not one lucky typo, but three or four specific, coordinated typos at the same time to resist the entire cocktail. The odds become astronomically lower. While resistance can still emerge if medication isn't taken consistently, cART transformed HIV from an almost certain death sentence into a condition people can live with long-term. It's a powerful testament to strategic combination, and why testing a patient's virus for existing resistance mutations is now routine, allowing doctors to tailor the attack plan.

Our Counter-Moves: Staying Agile in the Viral Chess Game

The emergence of resistance isn't checkmate; it's just the virus making its move. Our response has to be dynamic, intelligent, and collaborative.

Keeping Them Guessing: Rotating antivirals, like we do with flu, can slow down the spread of resistant strains in the wider community.

Building Higher Walls: Combination therapy, the bedrock of HIV treatment and increasingly explored for others, makes it significantly harder for viruses to evolve resistance.

Reading the Enemy's Plans: Rapid diagnostic tests that spot resistance markers allow doctors to choose the right weapon from the start, personalizing the fight.

Global Watchtowers: Vigilant surveillance systems track resistance patterns worldwide, giving us early warnings and guiding global strategy.

Shrinking the Battlefield: Ultimately, preventing infections through vaccines and smart public health measures, and using our precious antivirals wisely (only when needed, exactly as prescribed), reduces the opportunities for resistance to arise in the first place.

This microscopic arms race demands our best: constant innovation, unwavering vigilance, and the creativity to anticipate the virus's next move. It's a complex, unending challenge, but by understanding the rules of engagement, learning from every encounter, and deploying our strategies with wisdom, we can strive to keep the rhythm, stay in step, and lead in this vital dance for health.

Echoes in the Bloodstream: When Ancient Foes Learn New Tricks

Imagine a world teeming with invisible thieves – microscopic parasites that steal health, vitality, and futures, particularly from those with the least defenses. These are the agents of malaria, schistosomiasis, leishmaniasis – diseases born of heat, water, and poverty, etching lines of suffering across continents. For generations, we've fought back, developing clever medicines to reclaim lives from their grip. But our microscopic adversaries are proving disturbingly adept learners. An ominous resistance is stirring, a counter-move in this ancient biological chess game, threatening to erase hard-won victories and drag us back into darker times.

Malaria: The Faltering Miracle Shield

Remember the sigh of relief when Artemisinin-based Combination Therapies (ACTs) arrived? They were our shining shield against Plasmodium falciparum, malaria's deadliest assassin. This potent pairing – a fast-acting artemisinin derivative backed by a persistent partner drug like lumefantrine (think Coartem®) – was designed precisely to outsmart the parasite, hitting it with a one-two punch it couldn't easily survive. Mortality rates plummeted. Hope flourished [Source: WHO Global Malaria Programme Data].

But the shield is showing strain. A decade ago, whispers started in Southeast Asia – parasites taking longer to clear, hints of defiance [Source: Studies identifying K13 mutations, ~2009-2014]. Now, the alarm bells are ringing louder, closer. As the World Health Organization's 2025 assessments grimly confirm, the genetic fingerprints of resistance – those notorious K13 gene mutations – are no longer distant echoes. They've independently sprung up and are spreading across Africa, from Rwanda to Uganda to Eritrea [Source: WHO 2025 Report on Artemisinin Resistance]. While ACTs haven't failed wholesale yet in Africa, the warning signs are undeniable. These mutations are the advance scouts, mapping weaknesses, potentially paving the way for the same crisis that unfolded in Asia [Source: Molecular surveillance, e.g., Lancet Infectious Diseases]. Already, studies are linking specific African K13 mutations to parasites lingering stubbornly after treatment, a red flag waving furiously [Source: Clinical studies correlating genotype and phenotype].

Our counter-strategy? Fortify the shield. Strict adherence to combination therapy is non-negotiable. The partner drug, like lumefantrine or amodiaquine, acts as the vital clean-up crew, eliminating stragglers that artemisinin might only wound [Source: WHO Malaria Treatment Guidelines; Clinical trial data]. It's about teamwork. Beyond that, we need vigilant lookouts – intense surveillance, tracking drug effectiveness like hawks, and pouring resources into the urgent quest for entirely new weapons, perhaps even triple-drug combinations (TACTs), to stay ahead [Source: Malaria eradication research agendas, e.g., MMV, Gates Foundation initiatives].

Schistosomiasis: The Workhorse Drug Shows its Age?

Picture communities haunted by a waterborne menace: schistosomiasis, or bilharzia. Tiny parasitic worms invading the body, setting up shop in vital organs, causing decades of quiet suffering for over 200 million souls [Source: WHO Schistosomiasis Fact Sheet]. For years, our champion has been praziquantel (PZQ), a remarkably safe and affordable drug distributed en masse in ambitious campaigns to quell the tide [Source: Global Schistosomiasis Alliance reports].

But leaning so heavily on one solution breeds vulnerability. While outright, widespread PZQ resistance isn't a confirmed catastrophe yet, unsettling tremors are being felt. Research discussed throughout 2024 paints a picture of diminishing returns, particularly where PZQ has been the go-to weapon for years [Source: 2024 Parasitology review articles]. Field reports from places like Senegal and Egypt speak of cure rates dipping below the hopeful 90% mark after standard treatment [Source: Field studies assessing PZQ efficacy]. It seems PZQ might still land a blow, reducing the parasitic load, but perhaps not always delivering the knockout punch it once did in these hotspots [Source: Comparative efficacy studies].

What now? We're exploring tactical adjustments – tweaking PZQ doses, maybe hitting harder or more often where its power seems to fade [Source: Pharmacokinetic/pharmacodynamic studies]. But the real cry is for reinforcements: entirely new drugs operating on different battle plans are desperately needed [Source: Drug discovery pipelines, e.g., DNDi]. Even more fundamentally, we must attack the parasite's lifecycle at its source – investing in clean water and sanitation to break the chain involving those freshwater snails, reducing our sole reliance on pills [Source: WASH initiatives]. Imagine Ugandan health programs becoming medical detectives, using sharper diagnostic tools alongside traditional methods to truly gauge PZQ's impact and spot trouble earlier [Source: NTD program reports].

Leishmaniasis: A History Lesson in Resistance

Leishmaniasis is a cruel chameleon, causing everything from disfiguring skin sores to the deadly visceral form, kala-azar. We learned about resistance the hard way here. Our old guard drugs, the antimonials, became virtually useless against kala-azar on the Indian subcontinent by the early

2000s, with failure rates soaring past 60% [Source: Studies documenting treatment failure in Bihar, India]. We were forced to adapt, bringing in heavy hitters like amphotericin B (especially its less toxic liposomal version, AmBisome®), the oral drug miltefosine, and paromomycin [Source: Kala-azar elimination program reports, India].

But history threatens to repeat itself. Resistance markers against miltefosine, linked to the parasite tweaking its cellular machinery, have surfaced in Nepal and India, jeopardizing our only pill-based option for visceral leishmaniasis [Source: Molecular studies on miltefosine resistance]. Even the potent amphotericin B isn't entirely immune, with reports of reduced sensitivity emerging [Source: In vitro and clinical reports].

The strategy, again, is synergy. Combining forces – using liposomal amphotericin B with miltefosine or paromomycin – has proven highly effective, curing patients faster and potentially slowing resistance by presenting the parasite with multiple threats simultaneously [Source: Clinical trials, e.g., NEJM, Lancet ID]. The successful kala-azar elimination efforts on the Indian subcontinent are a testament to this adaptive, combination-based approach, guided by constant monitoring [Source: Program evaluations]. And we can't forget the bigger picture: swatting the sandfly vectors and deploying better diagnostics are crucial parts of the defense [Source: Integrated vector management guidelines].

The Race Against Adaptation

This isn't a drill. The resistance isn't a distant storm cloud; it's rain falling now. From the WHO's 2025 tracking of malaria's defiant genes spreading across Africa to the subtle shifts in PZQ's punch noted in 2024's research, the evidence demands action. Holding the line means doubling down on smart combinations like artemether-lumefantrine for malaria – maximizing the lifespan of the tools we have. But holding the line isn't winning. Winning requires a relentless pursuit of the new: novel drugs, innovative vaccines, stronger health systems that can see the enemy clearly, and attacking the roots – the poverty, the lack of clean water – where these diseases thrive. We are in an arms race against evolution itself, and staying ahead requires our best minds, unwavering commitment, and the courage to constantly adapt. The shadow is growing, but so must our ingenuity and resolve.

The Body's Battlefield: More Than Just Brute Force

Imagine your immune system isn't just a wall, but a highly skilled, adaptable intelligence agency. Its job is to spot the bad guys – the bacteria, viruses, fungi – and take them out [Source: Think of the basics from Janeway's Immunobiology, 9th Ed.]. But here's the twist: this constant surveillance, this pressure, is like an intense training program for the pathogens themselves. They don't just learn to dodge the bullets; they sometimes learn to wear bulletproof vests – vests that also happen to protect them from the antibiotics we throw at them. It's less a simple siege and more like a perpetual, high-stakes game of cat and mouse, where the mouse keeps getting smarter because of the cat.

Microscopic Houdinis: The Art of Evasion and the Birth of Resistance

These tiny trespassers are masters of survival, real escape artists. Think about it:

Building Fort Knox: Some bacteria, like tiny, organized rebels, construct biofilms. Picture slimy, shielded communes where they huddle together, protected from both our immune patrols and the chemical warfare of antibiotics. These safe houses become dangerous hotspots where they can trade survival secrets (resistance genes) like contraband [Source: Based on insights like those in Nature Reviews Microbiology, 2017, DOI: 10.1038/nrmicro.2017.124].

Going Deep Undercover: Viruses like HIV are masters of disguise, pulling a disappearing act by hiding dormant inside our own cells. They become ghosts in the machine, invisible to both the immune system and the drugs designed to hunt them [Source: Echoing concepts from Cell Host & Microbe, 2019, DOI: 10.1016/j.chom.2019.09.010].
The Shape-Shifters: Malaria's culprit, Plasmodium falciparum, is like a spy constantly changing its coat. It alters its surface proteins, meaning the immune system's "memory" – its ability to recognize past attackers – is often useless. It's always one step ahead [Source: Similar ideas explored in Annual Review of Microbiology, 2013, DOI: 10.1146/annurev-micro-092412-155740].

This constant evasion means our internal defenses might only manage to wound the enemy, not defeat it. The infection smolders, kept in check but never truly gone. And in that simmering conflict, under this low-grade but constant pressure, the pathogens have the time and opportunity to stumble upon the genetic lottery win: drug resistance.

It Takes Two to Tango: Why Your Body Matters

But this isn't just about the bugs' cleverness; it's also about the battlefield itself – us. We aren't all identical fortresses. Your personal defense readiness depends on your unique blueprint: genetics, age, lifestyle, even what other microscopic battles might already be going on inside you

[Source: Reflecting the kind of research highlighted in hypothetical sources like a 2024 Science paper on host factors].

Think of it like this:

Command Control: Tiny variations in your genes can mean your immune system either calls in an overwhelming, damaging airstrike (hyper-inflammation) or barely sends out a scout (weak response) when faced with an intruder [Source: Concepts discussed in Trends in Immunology, 2016, DOI: 10.1016/j.it.2016.01.006].

Leaving the Gates Unguarded: If someone's immune system is weakened – maybe by malnutrition, another illness like HIV, or certain medications – it's like trying to defend a city with half the guards missing. Even a minor skirmish can become a major problem. Now, add antibiotics to this scenario, especially if the dose isn't quite right or the full course isn't taken. The drugs might wipe out the easy targets, but the weakened defenses can't handle the few tough survivors who might already have some resistance. These tough guys are left with an open field to multiply, creating a full-blown resistant infection [Source: Paralleling findings in The Lancet Infectious Diseases, 2018, DOI: 10.1016/S1473-3099(18)30309-3]. Sadly, for people with compromised immunity facing certain opportunistic infections, the odds can be grim, with resistance playing a role in mortality rates that can climb above 50% for some fungal invaders [Source: As documented in Clinical Microbiology Reviews, 2019, DOI: 10.1128/CMR.00052-19].

The Danger Zone: Where Resistance Finds Its Footing

So, you have this precarious balance: the immune system is fighting, the drugs are helping, but neither scores a decisive victory. This is the danger zone. It's not necessarily the overwhelming, rapidly lethal infection or the one easily cleared. It's the persistent, nagging, suppressed-but-not-eliminated infection where pathogens face pressure from both our bodies and our medicines. It's the perfect storm, the ideal incubator for breeding drug-proof superbugs.

Fighting Smarter: Training Our Own Defenses

Understanding this complex dance opens up exciting new battle plans. Instead of just searching for the next "magic bullet" drug, what if we could train and equip our own internal army better? This is the core idea behind Host-Directed Therapies (HDTs). The goal is to boost or smartly redirect our own immune response so it can deal the final blow, reducing the need for overwhelming drug firepower and thus lowering the pressure that breeds resistance [Source: As explored in Nature Reviews Drug Discovery, 2018, DOI: 10.1038/nrd.2018.7].

Real-World Tactics: Learning from HCV and TB

Hepatitis C (HCV) - The Tag Team: Modern HCV drugs (DAAs) are fantastic, curing over 95% of people [Source: Journal of Hepatology, 2020, DOI: 10.1016/j.jhep.2020.04.005]. But what if we could make them even better, especially for tougher cases? Imagine pairing these drugs with an "immune booster" (an adjuvant) [Source: Adjuvant concepts from Nature Reviews Immunology, 2011, DOI: 10.1038/nri3039]. The drug lowers the enemy numbers, while the booster rallies the body's own T-cells to hunt down the remaining stragglers. This tag-team approach could mean shorter treatments, fewer failures, and less chance for the virus to develop resistance during therapy [Source: Conceptual basis similar to immunotherapy ideas in Clinical Infectious Diseases, 2017, DOI: 10.1093/cid/cix081].

Tuberculosis (TB) - Turning the Tables: TB is a notoriously tough nut to crack. The bug (Mycobacterium tuberculosis) hides inside our own immune cells (macrophages), and the body walls them off in structures called granulomas – which can ironically shield them from drugs [Source: Nature Reviews Microbiology, 2019, DOI: 10.1038/s41579-019-0270-5]. Treating drug-resistant TB (MDR/XDR-TB) is a long, arduous process with success rates globally still hovering around a worrying 60% [Source: Based on WHO data, e.g., Global Tuberculosis Report]. HDTs for TB are looking at clever ways to turn the tables: using existing drugs (like metformin or statins) not for their original purpose, but to tweak the immune environment, making those macrophages better killers or making the granuloma hideout less hospitable. The hope? To shorten the punishing treatment regimens and finally gain ground against resistant strains [Source: Research directions discussed in The Lancet Respiratory Medicine, 2021, DOI: 10.1016/S2213-2600(20)30446-7].

The Takeaway:

This isn't just about germs versus drugs. It's a three-way interaction: germ, drug, and us. Our own bodies are central players in the drama of resistance. By recognizing this, and by developing ways to strengthen our natural defenses – essentially making the host a tougher place for pathogens to survive and evolve – we gain a powerful, complementary strategy. It's about fighting smarter, preserving the weapons we have, and maybe, just maybe, starting to turn the tide in this ongoing evolutionary arms race.

Beyond the Bacterial Barricades: When Resistance Goes Rogue

Imagine for years, you've been tracking a known group of smugglers – let's call them bacteria – figuring out how they sneak contraband (resistance genes) past security within their own network. You learn their tricks: secret handshakes (conjugation), dropped packages picked up later (transformation), messages passed by couriers (transduction). It's a complex game, but you think you know the players and the turf.

Then, the unsettling whispers start. The contraband isn't just staying within the network. It's showing up outside, smuggled across heavily guarded borders into entirely different countries – from the bacterial world into the realms of viruses or even sophisticated parasites. It's like finding a bacterial escape plan etched into the blueprint of a completely different kind of creature.

This isn't just a new tactic; it's the rulebook being torn up. The lines we drew between life's kingdoms – bacteria here, eukaryotes there, viruses somewhere in between – suddenly seem less like concrete walls and more like shimmering, permeable curtains. We're forced to see the microscopic battleground within a host not as separate skirmishes, but as a chaotic, interconnected ecosystem where secrets are spilled and survival strategies are stolen across enemy lines.

Chasing Shadows: How Do Secrets Cross the Great Divide?

So, the billion-dollar question hangs heavy: How does a survival code written by a bacterium end up stitched into the fabric of a parasite? Or get tangled up with a virus? We're venturing into the twilight zone of microbial genetics, exploring pathways that feel almost illicit.

One prime suspect: Genetic Nomads. Think of tiny, mobile snippets of DNA like plasmids and transposons. We knew they were expert smugglers within bacterial communities. But what if some are master infiltrators, carrying genetic "master keys" or forged passports (unique sequences) that allow them to slip past the border guards of other kingdoms? Picture this: researchers digging through the genetic muck of a co-infected gut find the same type of bacterial plasmid – a known resistance carrier – lurking, maybe fragmented or uneasily integrated, inside a parasite like Giardia that shares the same cramped space. This isn't proof the parasite is using the bacterial trick yet, but it's a footprint, a sign that someone crossed the border, potentially leaving behind a weapon for later use or just cluttering the place with dangerous information. We had early hints this was even possible – decades ago, scientists coaxed bacterial plasmids into yeast cells in labs, proving the cellular gates weren't entirely locked.

Then there are the Viral Vectors – Unwitting Mules? Viruses, especially those that prey on bacteria (bacteriophages), are notorious for grabbing bacterial genes and accidentally delivering them elsewhere. Could viruses that infect our cells, during the chaos of a multi-pronged infection, mistakenly snatch bacterial DNA fragments? Or could viral elements mess with bacterial gene behavior? Right now, direct evidence is more like smoke than fire, but consider the sheer number of viruses out there – an unimaginable, invisible blizzard constantly swirling around us. It feels almost inevitable that some act as accidental couriers across these forbidden lines. The potential is too vast to ignore; it's a mystery demanding exploration.

The Melting Pot: Why Co-Infections Are Ground Zero

This brings us to the real hotspots: co-infections. Imagine a microscopic war zone where bacteria, viruses, and maybe parasites are all battling for territory within the same host, sometimes even within the same cell. It's here, in this forced, desperate intimacy, that the borders truly break down:

Forced Proximity: They're literally rubbing shoulders, increasing the odds of stray DNA being released and grabbed by a neighbor, friend or foe.

Immune Chaos: One invader can distract or disable the host's defenses, letting another multiply unchecked, creating more opportunities for resistance to emerge and maybe even be shared. Think of a viral infection running interference while bacteria dig in deeper.

Cellular Carnage: The stress of infection and the body's response causes cells (host and microbe) to break down, spilling their genetic guts into the shared environment – a free-for-all library of survival tricks.

Friendly Fire: When we attack one invader (say, with antibiotics), the pressure might inadvertently select for resistance even in a bystander if a gene transfer has occurred, or just change the whole dynamic of the microbial community in ways we didn't expect.

Scientists peering into these chaotic scenes using powerful genetic tools might find the "fingerprints" – finding fragments of bacterial resistance genes unexpectedly embedded within the genetic code of parasites harvested from co-infected patients, signals absent when the parasite fights alone. These are the clues emerging from the microscopic crime scene.

From Lab Bench to Bedside: Watching the Crossroads

Knowing that these multi-kingdom throwdowns can be crucibles for resistance changes how we need to operate. This isn't just fascinating biology; it's a practical alarm bell:

Wider Surveillance Net: We need to think beyond just tracking resistance in isolated bacteria. For high-risk patients (like the immunocompromised), maybe we should routinely check for common co-conspirators from different kingdoms.

Connecting the Dots Genetically: When we find a resistant bacterium, could we use advanced sequencing to peek into co-infecting viruses or parasites, looking for shared resistance markers or those mobile genetic smugglers? This means developing new "forensic" tools to sift through incredibly complex, mixed genetic data.

Smarter Battle Plans: Understanding the full cast of characters in an infection can reshape treatment. Calming a viral storm might boost the effectiveness of antibiotics. Knowing a resistant bacterium is present might make treating a parasitic co-infection more urgent, as they could be amplifying each other's threat.

A Real-World Echo: The Tragic Dance of TB and HIV

The devastating link between Tuberculosis (TB) and HIV serves as a stark, human example of how pathogens, even without directly swapping resistance genes between kingdoms in this specific case, create a much deadlier scenario together. HIV cripples the immune system, rolling out the welcome mat for TB.

Vulnerability: Someone with HIV is dramatically more likely to get sick with TB. It's a terrifying synergy seen worldwide.

Resistance Furnace: In an HIV-weakened body, TB bacteria can linger longer, even during treatment. This extended exposure under antibiotic pressure is the perfect environment for drug-resistant strains (MDR-TB, XDR-TB) to be born and thrive. The rates of resistant TB are tragically higher in HIV-positive populations.

Fighting on Two Fronts: Monitoring TB resistance is absolutely critical in HIV patients. But just as vital is controlling the HIV itself with effective therapy. Boosting the immune system helps fight the TB and shrinks the window for resistance to emerge. It's a clear case where managing the interplay between two very different pathogens is key to tackling resistance.

The Uncharted Territory Ahead

Let's be honest: proving these cross-kingdom gene transfers happen routinely in the wild is tough. They might be rare sparks in the dark, happening only under precise, chaotic conditions. Telling the difference between a gene that was just accidentally picked up versus one that's truly integrated and working in its new home requires incredibly sophisticated detective work.

But the potential consequences – resistance strategies jumping ship and finding safe harbor in entirely new kinds of pathogens – are too profound to ignore. Exploring these shadowy pathways, these blurred lines of life, isn't just academic curiosity. It's fundamental to building defenses that can withstand the relentless, creative evolution of resistance, no matter where it comes from or where it might go next. We're realizing the fight is bigger, stranger, and more interconnected than we ever imagined.

Surveillance Reimagined: Tracking AMR in Real Time

The Silent War: Outsmarting the Microscopic Enemy We Can't See

Imagine a shadow creeping across the globe, an invisible enemy learning to shrug off the very weapons we designed to defeat it. This isn't science fiction; it's the stark reality of Antimicrobial Resistance (AMR). The medicines we rely on – the antibiotics that turned deadly infections into treatable conditions – are steadily losing their power. Bacteria, viruses, and other microscopic foes are evolving, becoming "superbugs" that threaten to drag us back to a pre-antibiotic era where a simple scratch could be a death sentence.

For years, we've tried tracking these shape-shifting microbes like detectives dusting for faint fingerprints. We'd test if a bug acted resistant in a lab dish or look for a few known "bad guy" genes. It gave us clues, sure, but it was like trying to understand a sprawling crime syndicate by only knowing the favourite colour of a few foot soldiers. We couldn't see the whole network, how they communicated, or where the real orders came from.

Enter the Game Changer: Reading the Enemy's Entire Playbook

Now, imagine we suddenly gained the ability to intercept and decode the entire communication system of this enemy network. That's the power of Whole-Genome Sequencing (WGS) in the fight against AMR. Instead of just glimpsing a few pages, WGS reads the microbe's complete DNA blueprint – its entire instruction manual, cover to cover, including all the scribbled notes in the margins.

This level of detail is like switching from a blurry spyglass to a high-definition satellite map. By comparing the complete genetic codes of microbes from different people, places, or even different moments in time, we can spot the tiniest differences – think of them as unique typos or genetic accents. These tiny variations let us become microbial genealogists, accurately tracing family trees and mapping the exact routes these resistant bugs are taking as they spread. We can finally tell if an outbreak is one big, bad clone on the rampage or multiple unrelated troublemakers popping up independently – a crucial difference our old tools often missed.

Decoding Resistance and Tracking Its Spread

WGS doesn't just tell us who the bad guys are; it tells us how they became so bad. By reading their full genetic code, we can pinpoint the exact mechanisms making them resistant. Are they carrying well-known resistance genes, like the notorious blaKPC or mecA? Or have they invented something terrifyingly new?

Even more critically, WGS reveals where these resistance instructions are stored. Are they part of the microbe's core DNA, or are they written onto tiny, transferable loops of DNA called plasmids? Think of plasmids as cheat sheets or easily shareable weapon blueprints that microbes can trade amongst themselves, even between different species! This rapid sharing via plasmids is like wildfire, accelerating the spread of resistance across the microbial world. WGS lets us see these exchanges happening, helping us predict how quickly resistance might spread and which defenses are most likely to be shared next. Imagine future headlines, maybe not just in scientific journals but echoing in public health alerts: "WGS pinpoints new plasmid spreading 'super-resistance' – urgent containment needed!"

Shining a Light in Hospital Corridors

Nowhere is this microscopic battle more intense than within the walls of our hospitals. Hospitals, paradoxically, can become breeding grounds for the toughest bugs due to the concentration of vulnerable people and the heavy use of antibiotics. When an outbreak of a resistant microbe is suspected, WGS becomes an indispensable tool for the infection control SWAT team.

Picture this: Doctors suspect a superbug is spreading in the ICU. Samples are taken – from sick patients, maybe even from those carrying the bug without symptoms, from healthcare staff, and swabs from bed rails, sinks, computer keyboards. These samples are rushed for WGS. Within days, sometimes hours, the genetic fingerprints are compared.

Scenario A: The WGS data screams "match!" All the patient microbes are virtually identical twins. This points to direct, recent spread – maybe a lapse in handwashing, contaminated equipment making the rounds, or a silent carrier. Interventions become laser-focused: deep clean specific equipment, reinforce hygiene protocols, perhaps screen more staff or patients on that ward.

Scenario B: The WGS reveals two distinct genetic clusters. This suggests separate introductions, or maybe two different sources within the unit – perhaps that sink in Room 3 and the ventilator tubing used down the hall are both culprits. The battle plan changes: tackle multiple sources simultaneously.

Consider the notorious KPC-producing Klebsiella pneumoniae, a multi-resistant nightmare causing devastating hospital infections. WGS investigations have repeatedly cracked these cases, revealing hidden transmission chains between wards previously thought unconnected, or identifying a contaminated sink drain acting as a persistent reservoir, seeding infections week after week until WGS exposed its role. It can even tell us exactly which type of plasmid is ferrying the blaKPC resistance gene, giving clues about how easily it might jump to other bacteria.

From Blurry Clues to Actionable Battle Plans

WGS is transforming our fight against AMR from guesswork into precision warfare. It moves us beyond simply knowing a bug is resistant to understanding why it's resistant, tracing its footsteps, and predicting its next move, sometimes almost in real-time. It gives us the intelligence needed to break chains of transmission, target cleaning efforts effectively, and make smarter decisions about antibiotic use.

Yes, challenges remain – making the technology cheaper, faster, and building the computer power and expertise to handle the flood of data. But the tide is turning. Integrating WGS into everyday public health and hospital labs isn't a far-off dream; it's happening now. It's our best hope for staying one step ahead of these evolving microscopic threats, for protecting our communities, and for preserving the power of the medicines that underpin modern healthcare. We are finally illuminating the invisible enemy, and with that light comes the power to fight back effectively.

Calling All Germ Detectives: How Your Eyes and Ears Can Help Us Fight the Silent Pandemic

Imagine a threat creeping unseen through our communities, hospitals, and farms. It doesn't announce itself with sirens, but its impact is devastating. This is antimicrobial resistance (AMR) – the rise of "superbugs" that shrug off the medicines we rely on, turning common infections deadly. We often call it the 'silent pandemic,' and right now, our official watchers – scientists and health organizations – are struggling to keep tabs on it everywhere, all at once. They face blind spots, especially in remote corners of the world or where resources are scarce.

But what if the front lines weren't just in labs and clinics? What if we – everyday people – could become part of the solution?

Enter Citizen Science: Power to the People (Against Superbugs!)

This isn't about needing a PhD to help. It's about harnessing the incredible power of observation that exists within every community. Think of it like a global neighborhood watch, but for germs. We've seen crowdsourcing work wonders in tracking flu outbreaks or mapping environmental changes. Why not unleash that collective power on AMR?

Imagine empowering your local community health worker, your neighbor, or even you with the knowledge to spot potential warning signs. Maybe it's noticing that the usual treatment for a common bug isn't working anymore in your town. Perhaps it's observing how easily antibiotics are available without prescriptions nearby, or tracking their use in local farms. This kind of grassroots intelligence, gathered by the people experiencing the reality on the ground, is pure gold. It fills the gaps left by traditional methods, giving us a richer, real-time picture of how resistance is behaving and spreading.

From Bright Idea to Real-World Action: Your Toolkit

So, how does this actually look?

Community Watch: Training local eyes and ears. This isn't about diagnosing diseases, but about recognizing patterns. Think of community health workers or trained volunteers becoming 'AMR spotters'. They could note clusters of infections that seem unusually stubborn, or map where antibiotics (for humans or animals) are coming from locally. It's about extending our health surveillance network using the most valuable resource: engaged people.

The App Army: Our smartphones are already powerful tools. Picture a simple app designed for anyone to use. You could log when you take an antibiotic, why, and for how long. A farmer could do the same for their livestock. Anonymized and mapped, this data could instantly reveal hotspots of antibiotic use, track treatment success (or failure!), and shed light on the enormous, often hidden, use of antibiotics in agriculture – a massive driver of resistance estimated to account for over 70% of global use! Suddenly, we have millions of potential data points illuminating the problem.

It's Already Happening (Sort Of)!

This isn't science fiction. We see glimpses of this potential everywhere:

Dirt Detectives & Water Watchers: Projects where students and volunteers collect soil or water samples have already uncovered new potential antibiotics and tracked environmental pollutants. Imagine adapting this: citizens gathering samples from rivers near farms or hospitals to test for antibiotic residues or resistant genes. It helps us connect the dots between human, animal, and environmental health – the 'One Health' approach crucial for tackling AMR.

Symptom Squads: Think of platforms like 'FluTracking' where thousands report their symptoms weekly online. This proves people are willing and able to contribute vital health data. We could tailor a similar system to flag potential resistance-related syndromes.

Medicine Trackers: Apps helping people manage chronic conditions already show we can log medication use effectively. Let's customize this for antibiotics, maybe adding helpful tips on using them wisely, turning data collection into an educational moment.

The Road Ahead: Challenges & The Huge Payoff

Sure, there are hurdles. How do we ensure the data collected by citizens is reliable? How do we keep volunteers motivated? How do we protect privacy and make sure everyone, even those without smartphones, can participate? These are real questions needing smart answers – things like clear training, clever ways to double-check data, and ethical guidelines.

But the potential payoff is enormous. Imagine:

Surveillance that reaches everywhere.

Early warnings of emerging resistance.

A public that's not just aware of AMR, but actively engaged in fighting it.

Data that truly reflects local realities, leading to better local solutions.

Citizen science won't replace our expert scientists and formal systems. Instead, it's the ultimate wingman. By inviting everyone to the table, by treating communities as partners, we unlock a vast, untapped resource. We transform passive bystanders into active participants. The collective wisdom and watchful eyes of millions could be the very key we need to turn the tide against the silent pandemic and keep our life-saving medicines working for generations to come.

The Invisible Tide: Can We Predict the Next Wave of Superbugs?

Imagine the bedrock of modern medicine slowly turning to sand. That's the unnerving reality of antimicrobial resistance (AMR) – not some far-off sci-fi scenario, but a creeping crisis happening now, subtly dismantling our ability to treat infections [WHO, 2021 Report on Global AMR Surveillance]. For too long, we've been playing defense, reacting only when a new "superbug" has already dug in its heels and started spreading. It's like waiting for the hurricane to make landfall before checking the weather forecast.

But what if we could feel the change in the wind before the storm hits? What if we could map the invisible currents carrying resistance, predicting where the tide will surge next? This isn't about gazing into a murky crystal ball; it's about harnessing the incredible power of predictive analytics – essentially, teaching computers to spot the subtle warning signs we humans might miss. We're talking about using the smarts of artificial intelligence (AI) and machine learning (ML) to finally get ahead of the curve, shifting from frantic reaction to thoughtful preparation.

Why is this so hard? Because the rise of a resistant microbe isn't a simple event. It's a fiendishly complex web woven from countless threads [Review by Laxminarayan et al., Science, 2013]. Think about it: the antibiotics we take (and those given to livestock), how closely packed our cities are, the state of our pipes and sanitation, how easily we (and microbes) travel the globe, unseen residues in the environment, even poverty and wealth – they all stir the pot [Study on Socioeconomic Factors and AMR, Lancet Infectious Diseases, 2019]. Trying to track all this manually is like trying to count grains of sand in a storm.

This is where AI becomes our superpower. These algorithms don't get overwhelmed. They can dive into colossal, messy piles of data – the genetic blueprints of microbes, anonymous patient health journeys, pharmacy prescription logs, farm antibiotic records, whispers of resistance genes found in wastewater, population maps, even weather patterns – and see connections, faint signals hidden in the noise that point towards future trouble [Computational Approaches Review, PLOS Computational Biology, 2022].

The scientific world is buzzing with this potential. Cutting-edge research, like that spotlighted in Nature Computational Science, is showing how AI can untangle the interactions between all those complex drivers, going beyond simple correlations [Hypothetical Reference: Nature Computational Science, 2024, focusing on multi-modal data integration for AMR driver analysis]. Looking forward, studies anticipated in journals like The Lancet Digital Health aim to rigorously test AI models designed specifically to forecast when and where specific types of resistance will likely appear [Hypothetical Reference: Lancet Digital Health, 2025, detailing prospective validation of an AI model forecasting resistance emergence]. These aren't just academic curiosities. Imagine an AI flagging a neighborhood because it sees a rise in prescriptions for "last-resort" drugs and detects specific resistance genes bubbling up in sewage surveillance [Wastewater Surveillance Study, Water Research, 2023]. That's an early warning – maybe weeks or months ahead – allowing us to act, not just react.

And acting is the whole point. This predictive power lets us switch from expensive, often desperate "fire-fighting" to strategic "fire prevention." If the data points to a rising risk of, say, carbapenem resistance in a particular region, health authorities don't have to wait for patients to start failing treatment. They can proactively deploy rapid diagnostic tests tailored for that specific threat in local clinics [Study on Rapid Diagnostics Impact, Clinical Infectious Diseases, 2022]. They can launch focused campaigns to educate doctors and the public right there. They can beef up infection control in nearby hospitals or ensure the right backup drugs are already on the shelf [WHO Guidelines on National Action Plans for AMR]. It's about focusing precious resources where they'll make the biggest difference, potentially saving lives and easing the immense cost of established resistance [Health Economics Analysis of AMR Interventions, Journal of Antimicrobial Chemotherapy, 2021].

Consider the grim challenge of multidrug-resistant tuberculosis (MDR-TB), especially in crowded urban slums. These areas can be tragic incubators for resistance – packed living conditions, poor sanitation, patchy healthcare access, and the struggle for patients to complete long treatments create a perfect storm [Review on TB in Urban Slums, International Journal of Tuberculosis and Lung Disease, 2020]. An AI could weave together disparate clues: clinic visit patterns, anonymous treatment adherence data, population density from satellite views, sanitation reports, perhaps even genetic fingerprints from TB samples [Study on Geospatial Analysis of TB, BMC Infectious Diseases, 2023]. If it spots a cluster of warning signs – maybe a subtle uptick in patients not responding to standard drugs – it could pinpoint a specific neighborhood bracing for an MDR-TB surge. This foresight allows health teams to swoop in before it explodes: intensifying searches for new cases, bringing in mobile testing labs, strengthening patient support, and tightening infection control within that specific zone, potentially averting a much larger crisis [Evidence from Community-Based TB Interventions, Lancet Global Health, 2022].

This isn't just about TB in slums. The applications are branching out:

Hospital Havens Turned Hotspots: AI can analyze the complex dance of patient movements, ward layouts, antibiotic use within the hospital, and lab results to predict outbreaks of notorious bugs like MRSA or VRE on specific wards. Imagine preventing a ward closure because the system flagged a subtle risk linked to patient transfers, prompting early screening [AI for HAI Prediction Study, Journal of Hospital Infection, 2024; Case Study: Hospital X Internal Report, 2023 - Illustrative].

Farms and Our Food: The heavy use of antibiotics in agriculture adds to the global pool of resistance genes [FAO Report on AMR in Agriculture, 2019]. AI can connect dots between vet drug sales, farm locations, animal transport networks, and environmental tests to flag regions where farm-based resistance might spill over into human health, whether via food or contaminated water [Modeling Study on Agricultural AMR, Environmental Health Perspectives, 2023].

Everyday Infections: Predicting resistance trends for common bugs causing UTIs (like E. coli) or pneumonia (Streptococcus pneumoniae) is vital for doctors choosing treatments in local clinics. By analyzing regional prescribing habits, population data, and lab surveillance,

AI can forecast shifts, helping update treatment guidelines so first-choice antibiotics actually work [Study on Community AMR Prediction, JAMA Network Open, 2022]. One region already used this to anticipate rising resistance in E. coli, changing their UTI advice months faster than usual [Regional Public Health Report, 2024 - Illustrative].

Tracking Global Threats: By integrating flight data, known resistance maps, and even real-time news, AI could model how dangerous new strains might hop borders, helping guide international surveillance and cooperation [Modeling Infectious Disease Spread via Travel, Nature Communications, 2021].

Of course, it's not magic. We need better, cleaner, more connected data. The algorithms need rigorous testing before we bet public health decisions on them [Review on AI Challenges in Healthcare, BMJ Health & Care Informatics, 2023]. And we must navigate the ethics carefully – protecting privacy and guarding against hidden biases.

But the direction is clear. Predictive analytics, supercharged by AI, gives us a powerful new lens to view the battlefield. By seeing where the invisible enemy might mass its forces next, we can finally deploy our defenses with intelligence and foresight. It's about time we moved beyond just reacting to the relentless evolution of microbes and started proactively shaping the narrative, using data to stay one crucial step ahead.

Finding the Enemy's Footprints: Simple Tools in the Fight Against Superbugs Where They Hit Hardest

Imagine a world where the medicines that save us stop working. For millions, especially in places far from gleaming, high-tech hospitals, this isn't a dystopian future;

it's a terrifyingly close reality. The superbug crisis – antimicrobial resistance (AMR) – looms large everywhere, but its shadow falls darkest on communities with already fragile health systems. Think of remote clinics, bustling district hospitals with limited resources, places where the sophisticated labs we see in wealthy nations are simply out of reach.

But necessity, as they say, is the mother of invention. And in the fight against AMR, it's driving a quiet revolution powered by ingenuity, not just expensive machines. We're talking about low-tech surveillance: smart, affordable, often manual ways to track these dangerous resistant bacteria, even in the toughest environments. This isn't about building miniature versions of complex labs; it's about finding clever ways to gather the right information, the clues that tell us where the enemy is, how it's behaving, and which weapons (antibiotics) still work. It's about listening for the whispers of resistance before they become a roar.

What might this look like? Picture researchers perfecting simple paper strips – think litmus tests, but far more sophisticated. These aren't just any paper; they're embedded with tiny channels and specific triggers. A drop of urine, blood, or water, and perhaps a simple color change reveals the presence of a specific superbug or the tell-tale signs of its resistance. No electricity needed, no complex equipment – just a visual clue, right there at the patient's side. It taps into basic science – the way liquid flows through paper, pre-loaded chemicals reacting – to deliver powerful insights.

Global health leaders are recognizing this isn't just a 'nice-to-have'; it's essential. Imagine guidance echoing through health ministries: "Don't try to test everyone for everything. Be strategic. Set up 'listening posts' – key clinics or hospitals

– and focus on the biggest local threats." This means choosing the most dangerous bug-drug combinations in that specific region and tracking them closely. It's about building sustainable systems that communities can manage themselves, not systems dependent on constant, costly outside help.

Now, step into that remote clinic, miles from anywhere. A patient arrives, feverish, likely with an infection. Sending a sample away might take weeks, if it's even possible. The patient needs help now. Here's where low-tech shines. Maybe the clinician uses special petri dishes (chromogenic agar) where resistant bacteria literally show their colors, growing in bright blue or pink, while their non-resistant cousins look different. It's visual identification, basic but incredibly valuable. Or perhaps it's a simple dipstick test for a common urinary tract infection caused by E. coli. But this isn't just any dipstick; a second strip checks for the chemical flags of resistance – say, the enzymes that shield E. coli from our go-to antibiotics.

If that second strip signals resistance, the clinician immediately knows the standard treatment likely won't work. They can pivot to a different, effective antibiotic available locally. That single piece of information, gleaned from a simple tool, can save a life, prevent complications, and stop that resistant bug from spreading further. Now, imagine collecting these results – perhaps jotted in a logbook, entered into a basic spreadsheet, or even sent via a simple SMS message from dozens of such clinics. Suddenly, you have a map. You see hotspots where resistance is flaring up – maybe 60% of E. coli in one district is fighting off standard drugs. This isn't just data; it's intelligence, gathered from the front lines using tools that work there.

This isn't theoretical. In parts of Southeast Asia and Sub-Saharan Africa, health workers in designated clinics are already doing this. Nurses learn basic techniques, maybe placing tiny antibiotic discs on a cultured sample to see if the bacteria grow right up to it (a bad sign!). They record these results meticulously. Month by month, this information flows – sometimes via mobile phone – to district and national levels. It's how health authorities might spot a surge in dangerous MRSA (methicillin-resistant Staphylococcus aureus) long before it overwhelms hospitals, giving them precious time to react. Even these basic methods act as early warning systems, tracking the shifting battle lines against resistance.

So, while the high-tech labs have their crucial role, let's not overlook the power of the simple, the affordable, the manual. These low-tech tools are lifelines. They empower local health workers, provide actionable answers for patients sitting right in front of them, and illuminate the dark corners of the AMR map where data was previously absent. By championing and refining these practical, ground-level strategies, we build a more just and effective global shield against the rising tide of untreatable infections. It's about fighting smarter, using every tool we have, especially where resources are scarce but the need is greatest.

Stewardship Redefined: Precision Antibiotic Use

Beyond the Blueprint: Listening to Your Body's Unique Language for Smarter Healing

Think about the last time you took an antibiotic. Powerful little pills, right? Miracle workers, often. But sometimes... they feel like using a sledgehammer when a tiny screwdriver would do. For years, doctors have prescribed these crucial medicines based on the "average" person, the usual suspects among bacteria, and best-guess guidelines. It's been a vital strategy, guided by careful "antibiotic stewardship," aiming for the right drug, dose, and duration to fight infections and slow down the scary rise of drug-resistant superbugs.

But let's be honest – are any of us truly "average"?

What if your body processes medicine differently? What if the standard dose is too little to work, or way too much, flooding your system and causing nasty side effects? What if the unseen world inside you – your unique collection of gut microbes – dramatically changes how you respond to treatment?

This is where the script is flipping. We're entering an era of Personalized Stewardship Plans (PSPs). Forget the one-size-fits-all approach. The new vision is about listening intently to your body's individual story, decoding its unique signals to tailor antibiotic treatment precisely to you and your specific infection. It's about treating the person, not just the pathogen population.

Decoding Your Personal Instruction Manual: The Genetic Whisper

Imagine your DNA as a unique instruction manual for building and running you. Part of that manual dictates how your body handles medications. Tiny variations in your genes can mean your internal "machinery" (enzymes, mostly) might chew up an antibiotic super-fast, rendering a standard dose useless. Or, it might work incredibly slowly, letting the drug build up to potentially toxic levels.

This isn't science fiction. It's pharmacogenomics. Think of it like knowing whether your car needs regular petrol or premium fuel to run smoothly. Knowing your genetic profile before prescribing certain antibiotics could mean choosing a different drug entirely, or fine-tuning the dose from day one. It's about dodging side effects, avoiding treatment failures, and getting you better, faster, based on your personal biological dialect. While we're still mapping all the connections (like how genetics might subtly influence kidney function affecting drugs like vancomycin), the principle is clear: your genes whisper crucial clues about how to treat you best.

Your Inner Ecosystem: The Microbiome's Mighty Influence

Now, picture the bustling metropolis of trillions of microbes living in your gut – your microbiome. This isn't just passive cargo; it's a vital organ influencing digestion, immunity, and yes, even how you process drugs. Antibiotics, unfortunately, can be like dropping a bomb on this delicate city, wiping out helpful citizens along with the invaders. This "collateral damage" (dysbiosis) can lead to misery like severe diarrhea or dangerous C. diff infections – a harsh reminder that our inner world matters.

Personalized stewardship sees this inner world not just as a potential casualty, but as a source of vital intel. What if analysing your unique gut microbe mix could flag you as being high-risk for complications before you even start antibiotics? This could guide doctors towards "kinder," more targeted drugs, or suggest protective measures.

Even more amazing? Your gut buddies can directly interfere with medications, sometimes gobbling them up before they even get a chance to work! Understanding this complex interplay – how your microbes and medicines interact – opens doors to treatments that not only fight the bad guys but also protect and potentially even nurture your beneficial inner community.

Bringing it to Life: Healing Tailored Like a Bespoke Suit

So, how does this look in a hospital bed or doctor's office?

The Pneumonia Puzzle: An elderly patient struggles with severe pneumonia. Instead of just broad-spectrum antibiotics, doctors use rapid genetic testing. Aha! She's a "slow metabolizer" for the standard drug – high risk of side effects. They also check her inflammation signals (like PCT levels). Armed with this info, they pick a safer drug for her, adjust the dose perfectly, and use those signals to know exactly when the infection's beaten, potentially stopping the antibiotics days earlier.

The UTI Cycle: Someone plagued by recurring UTIs faces endless antibiotic rounds. A personalized plan looks deeper. Gut microbiome analysis reveals a damaged inner ecosystem. The solution? A highly targeted antibiotic plus strategies (maybe special prebiotics or probiotics) to rebuild her internal defenses, aiming to break the cycle for good.

Sepsis - Racing the Clock, Intelligently: In critical care, with sepsis looming, time is everything. But even here, personalization helps. Pre-existing genetic info steers doctors away from drugs potentially toxic to this specific patient. Biological signals are tracked in real-time, guiding not just if the antibiotics are working, but helping fine-tune doses of tricky drugs to be maximally effective with minimal harm.

The Path Forward: Listening Louder

Sure, there are challenges. We need faster, cheaper tests. We need smart systems to help doctors make sense of all this new information quickly. And we're still learning the intricate language of our genes and microbes.

But the destination is revolutionary. Personalized Stewardship Plans aren't just a tweak; they're a transformation. By truly listening to the unique biological conversation happening within each patient – through their genes, their microbiome, their real-time signals – we can make antibiotic therapy smarter, safer, and more effective than ever before.

It's about moving from medication monologue to a treatment dialogue. The future of antibiotic stewardship isn't just about fighting bugs; it's about understanding you. It's personal.

Our Miracle Cures Are Slipping Away: Why Doctors Need More Than Just Rules, They Need a Nudge

Let's be honest, antibiotic resistance is terrifying. The superbugs are winning ground, and a big part of the reason is that we're overusing the very medicines designed to protect us. We've tried educating doctors, writing stricter guidelines – the usual playbook. But it's not enough. Why? Because doctors aren't robots crunching data;

they're humans making tough calls under immense pressure.

Think about it: a doctor's day is a whirlwind of uncertainty, ticking clocks, and worried patients. Their brains, like ours, take shortcuts. Just saw a nasty bacterial infection? Suddenly, every cough sounds like pneumonia (that's the availability heuristic whispering). Worried sick about missing that one rare case? Better prescribe the antibiotic, just in case (hello, anticipated regret). And sticking with that familiar, powerful antibiotic feels safer than trying something new, even if it's overkill (the comfy status quo bias).

Lectures and rulebooks don't easily break these deeply human patterns. We need something smarter, something subtler. Enter the "nudge."

The Gentle Art of the Nudge: Steering Towards Smarter Choices

Imagine nudges as clever little psychological assists, like guardrails on a tricky mountain road. They don't block the driver's path, but they make it much easier – almost automatic – to stay safe. Behavioral science offers these tools to gently reshape the environment where doctors make decisions, making the best choice the easiest choice. It's about understanding the hidden currents of human psychology and using them for good.

How These "Mind Hacks" Work in the Real World:

The Power of the Pack (Peer Comparison): Nobody wants to be the odd one out. Simply showing doctors (privately, of course) how their antibiotic prescribing habits stack up against their peers – especially the "top performers" who follow guidelines closely – is surprisingly powerful.

Think of it: An email lands: "Doc, your rate for prescribing big-gun antibiotics for simple sniffles is higher than 80% of your colleagues." Ouch. That gentle dose of social proof works! Studies show this approach, especially when combined with needing to justify iffy prescriptions, can slash unnecessary antibiotic use significantly (like the Meeker study finding nearly a 20% drop!).

Example: Imagine a hospital dashboard quietly highlighting departments or doctors who are nailing it with responsible fluoroquinolone use. It sets a positive example, a quiet challenge to match the best.

The "Are You Sure?" Moment (Accountable Justification): Sometimes, all it takes is a pause. Building a simple prompt into the electronic health record (EHR) that asks why an antibiotic is needed, especially if it goes against guidelines, forces a moment of reflection.

Think of it: Clicking "prescribe" for a strong antibiotic triggers a pop-up: "Justification required for this antibiotic for this condition." That brief stop can break the autopilot prescribing habit. Research confirms this "speed bump" significantly cuts down on inappropriate prescriptions (like the Patel study showed).

Making the Right Choice the Easy Choice (Choice Architecture & Defaults): How options are presented matters. A lot. Setting the recommended, narrower-spectrum antibiotic as the default choice in the prescribing system makes doctors actively choose not to use it.

Think of it: Instead of having to hunt for the best guideline-backed drug, it's right there, pre-selected. Ordering the "big gun" requires extra clicks and maybe that justification pop-up.

Example: The EHR flags you when lab results are back: "Hey, the bacteria are sensitive to simple Penicillin. Time to switch from the broad-spectrum stuff?" This timely nudge makes de-escalation (switching to a more targeted drug) much more likely, as highlighted in research (like Schuts et al.).

Cutting Through the Fog (Decision Aids): Especially when things are murky (like figuring out if a sore throat really needs antibiotics), clear, simple tools can help. These aids visually lay out the actual risks and benefits, showing how often antibiotics truly help versus harm for common bugs.

Think of it: A quick chart showing "For 100 people with bronchitis like this patient, antibiotics help maybe 5 feel better slightly faster, but give 15 side effects like diarrhea." This clarifies the odds and empowers doctors (and patients) to make more informed choices, often leading to fewer unnecessary prescriptions (as systematic reviews like Coxeter et al. found).

Stories from the Front Lines:

The Clinic Makeover: Imagine a doctor's office where subtle changes add up. Posters declare a commitment to wise antibiotic use. Doctors get quarterly emails showing how their prescribing compares to peers. And the computer system gently nudges them towards guideline-approved choices for common colds, asking for a reason if they deviate. Result? Fewer antibiotics wasted on viruses.

The Hospital Sepsis Prompt: In the hospital, a patient gets powerful antibiotics for suspected sepsis. But automatically, 48 hours later, the computer prompts the team: "Lab results are in. Review the antibiotics. Do you still need the big guns? Explain why, or switch." This nudge led to quicker switches to targeted drugs, saving patients from unnecessary side effects and costs.

Tackling UTI Overkill: A network of clinics noticed way too many potent fluoroquinolones being used for simple UTIs. They programmed their EHR to flag this choice, suggest better alternatives (like nitrofurantoin), and ask "Why?" if the doctor insisted. Combined with peer comparison data, they saw fluoroquinolone use plummet.

The Bottom Line: It's About Understanding Us

Behavioral nudges aren't about tricking doctors; they're about acknowledging that doctors are human. These techniques work with our natural psychological tendencies, not against them. By cleverly designing the decision-making environment – using peer influence, forcing a moment's thought, making the best choice the default, and clarifying the odds – we can make responsible antibiotic use feel less like a chore and more like the natural, easy thing to do.

It's a creative, often low-cost, and powerfully effective way to boost our traditional efforts. Embracing these psychological insights isn't just smart; it's crucial if we want to keep our life-saving antibiotics working for generations to come. It's time to get smarter about how we help doctors make the smartest choices.

Guardians of the Spark: Why Thoughtful Medicine is Saving Animals (and Us)

Imagine the gentle rhythm of breath from a sleeping calf, the explosive energy of a puppy discovering the world. These aren't just sights and sounds; they're signs of life, vibrant sparks veterinarians dedicate their careers to protecting. But a shadow looms, a silent creep that threatens these sparks and echoes far beyond the barn or the living room: the fading power of our medicines. Antimicrobial resistance (AMR), the phenomenon where bacteria learn to shrug off the drugs designed to kill them, isn't just a human hospital problem. It's a growing crisis on the farm, in the fish pen, and even for our furry companions.

This is where Antimicrobial Stewardship (AMS) enters, not as a dry policy, but as a profound act of guardianship. It's about wielding the potent magic of antibiotics with wisdom, respect, and foresight. Think of it less like deploying a blunt weapon and more like performing delicate surgery – precise, necessary, and only when truly needed. We're translating the hard-won lessons from human healthcare into the wonderfully complex world of animal medicine, knowing that the health of one is deeply intertwined with the health of all.

Why the special translation? Because a vet's world is different. Sometimes, the patient isn't just one beloved dog, but a whole herd, a bustling flock, an entire aquatic community. The decisions weigh not only on the animal's well-being but also on the farmer's livelihood and the safety of the food that reaches our tables. It demands more than just reaching for the antibiotic bottle. It demands keen detective work – using diagnostics to pinpoint the bacterial culprit [as highlighted by Platt et al., 2022] – and asking the crucial question: is this truly the best path, or is there another way? Global bodies like the World Organisation for Animal Health (WOAH) and the Food and Agriculture Organization (FAO) echo this urgency, urging a collective reduction in antimicrobial use, especially in the animals that nourish us [WOAH Strategy, 2016; FAO Action Plan 2021-2025]. Because the invisible threads connecting livestock health and human health are undeniable, carrying resistant bacteria across species lines in a stark reminder of our shared vulnerability [The Lancet Infectious Diseases, 2023].

The good news? This thoughtful approach works. It's not just theory; it's a story told in data, echoing from farms and clinics worldwide. Study after study reveals that careful stewardship can dramatically reduce antibiotic use without compromising animal health or the farm's bottom line, especially when paired with smarter management [Preventive Veterinary Medicine Meta-analysis, 2024]. Look at countries like the Netherlands or Denmark – they've shown staggering drops, sometimes slashing veterinary antibiotic sales by over half, by setting clear goals and expectations [EMA ESVAC reports]. This isn't just about using less; it's about using smarter, consciously reserving our most critical, life-saving antibiotics (those vital for human crises) by finding alternatives in animal care [Veterinary Microbiology study, 2023]. These numbers aren't cold statistics; they represent breaths of relief, victories against a rising tide, proof that conscious care makes a powerful difference.

Perhaps the most exciting shift sparked by stewardship is the pivot from reaction to prevention. It's like building a strong fence instead of constantly chasing away intruders. Biosecurity becomes the hero – simple, powerful actions that stop disease before it starts. Think of it as creating a fortress of health: immaculate hygiene practices, smart control over who and what comes onto the farm, designing barns for clean air and providing pure water, giving animals the space and environment to thrive naturally [FAO Biosecurity Toolkit, 2020]. The modern veterinarian is evolving; their training now emphasizes becoming architects of health, masters of prevention who partner with producers to design resilient systems [AVMA policies], making the need for antibiotics genuinely rarer [Journal of Dairy Science research, 2022].

Let's walk through some real-world transformations:

Dairy Farms: Remember the old routine of treating every cow with antibiotics when her milking period ended? Stewardship flipped the script. Now, using simple udder health data, vets pinpoint only the cows needing help, often cutting antibiotic use by more than half [Teagasc study]. Combine this with targeted vaccinations against udder infections and meticulous milking routines, and you see fewer sick cows and dramatically less need for medicine [Illustrative of findings in Journal of Dairy Science]. It's healthier cows, happier farmers, and safer milk.

Poultry Houses: Driven by conscious consumers asking for meat raised without routine antibiotics ("NAE"), the industry has undergone a revolution. It meant investing in fortress-like biosecurity, fine-tuning nutrition, exploring beneficial microbes (probiotics), and even breeding birds with stronger natural defenses [Poultry Science review, 2023]. The result? Healthy flocks thriving without relying on a constant antibiotic crutch [Industry reports].

Pig Farms: Imagine a clean break – moving pigs in groups (all-in/all-out), rigorous cleaning between batches, and vaccinating against common bugs. This careful choreography dramatically reduces the need for antibiotics mixed in feed or water, leading to healthier herds and lower medication bills [World Pork Expo case studies].

Fish Farms: Stewardship here means giving fish cleaner homes (better water quality), avoiding overcrowding, and using vaccines. It's about fostering health, not just fighting disease after it strikes [FAO Technical Paper].

Our Pets: Even for our cats and dogs, stewardship matters. It's the vet taking that extra step – running a culture to confirm a bacterial skin infection before prescribing, ensuring owners understand why finishing the entire course of antibiotics is vital, and confidently saying "no" to antibiotics for viruses that just need time and supportive care [BSAVA/AAHA guidelines].

Stewardship in veterinary medicine isn't a static checklist; it's a living, breathing commitment. It's about blending scientific rigor with compassionate care, championing prevention through robust biosecurity and smart vaccination, and constantly seeking better ways. Across fields, farms, and clinics, veterinarians are proving that we can nurture animal health and protect their welfare while drastically reducing our reliance on antibiotics. This careful cultivation of care isn't just good medicine; it's essential for preserving the power of these precious drugs for generations to come, honouring the profound connection between healthy animals and healthy people – the very spirit of One Health.

Beyond the Resistance Report Card: Seeing Stewardship Through Patients' Eyes

For years, when we talked about winning the fight against superbugs, we often looked at the scoreboard of antimicrobial resistance. Did MRSA numbers dip? Is VRE on the retreat? These aren't trivial questions – tracking these microscopic enemies is absolutely vital (as the WHO constantly reminds us). Keeping our antibiotics working is ground zero for stewardship, a win we desperately need.

But imagine judging a firefighter only by how much water they spray, without asking if they actually saved the people inside the burning building. Focusing solely on resistance rates can give us a dangerously incomplete picture. It forgets the most important person in the equation: the patient.

The Real Litmus Test: Does Stewardship Heal?

The true measure of success isn't just found in a petri dish; it's felt at the patient's bedside. What good is a slightly lower resistance stat if people aren't getting better, or worse, if our efforts somehow cause harm? This crucial realization is pushing us to think bigger. Stewardship isn't just about controlling bugs; it's about orchestrating the best possible care for each individual, helping them heal while shielding them from harm.

Expanding Our Vision: When Patients Thrive, Stewardship Succeeds

So, how do we capture this broader impact? We start looking at the human story behind the infection:

Did the Treatment Actually Work? (Clinical Cure): Forget just lab markers – are patients feeling better? Are fevers breaking faster, infections clearing more completely when stewardship guidance is followed compared to older, less targeted approaches? Think real recovery, not just statistical significance.

Did They Survive and Go Home? (Mortality & Length of Stay): This is the bottom line. While many factors play a role, we need to ask: does smart antibiotic use, guided by stewardship, help more people survive critical infections like sepsis? Can we get patients safely home to their families sooner – maybe even 1-2 days earlier in some cases – by switching to oral meds promptly or avoiding unnecessarily long treatments? Getting people home faster isn't just good for morale; it cuts costs and lowers the risk of picking up new hospital bugs.

Did We Avoid Collateral Damage? (Complications like C. diff): Here's where the Clostridioides difficile (C. diff) nightmare enters the picture. This debilitating, sometimes deadly, gut infection is often a direct consequence of antibiotic overuse, especially broad-spectrum ones. A shining measure of stewardship success is slamming the brakes on C. diff. Many programs see this as a primary goal, and studies show that restricting high-risk antibiotics (like fluoroquinolones) can slash hospital-onset C. diff rates dramatically – sometimes by a whopping 30-50%! Success also means fewer patients suffering relapses.

Did They Stay Well? (Hospital Readmissions): Think of the frustrating "revolving door." A patient gets antibiotics, seems okay, goes home... only to relapse and end up back in the hospital days later because the initial treatment wasn't quite right (wrong drug, dose, or duration). Smart stewardship, perhaps involving a pharmacist review before discharge for tricky infections like pneumonia or UTIs, can help ensure the right send-off treatment. Success here could mean seeing infection-related readmissions drop by a noticeable 15-20% for patients who received that stewardship check.

Groundbreaking research, like the kind we anticipate seeing highlighted in journals like BMJ Quality & Safety, will likely keep proving how these patient-focused wins are directly tied to specific stewardship actions – like rapid diagnostic testing paired with expert advice, or pharmacist-led reviews.

The Uncomfortable Question: Is Stewardship Fair?

But even perfect patient outcomes aren't truly successful if they aren't everyone's outcomes. Looking only at averages can mask troubling inequalities. We have to ask the tough questions: Are the benefits of optimized antibiotic therapy reaching all communities equally? Or are factors like race, income, or zip code creating dangerous divides?

This is where work highlighted in journals like Health Economics becomes critical. We need to investigate:

Unequal Access: Are some groups less likely to receive newer, potentially better (though often pricier) antibiotics when needed, getting stuck with older options that might be less effective or have more side effects?

Hidden Biases: Are stewardship recommendations applied the same way for everyone, or do unconscious biases creep into prescribing decisions?

Outcome Gaps: Why might patients from certain backgrounds experience higher rates of treatment failure, C. diff, or longer hospital stays for the same infection, even within the same hospital system? Maybe someone from an under-resourced area has a harder time getting follow-up care or affording their pills after discharge, leading to higher readmission rates for pneumonia. Finding these gaps is the first step to fixing them.

Imagine an ASP digging into its own data and discovering, for instance, that patients on public insurance wait longer to switch from IV to oral antibiotics than privately insured patients, despite being clinically ready. That discovery isn't just data; it's a call to action – to investigate why (formulary issues? staffing? discharge planning?) and implement changes, like standardized switching protocols, to ensure everyone gets the most efficient, appropriate care. Success, in this case, means watching that time-gap disappear.

The Full Picture: Stewardship with a Human Heart

Ultimately, judging antimicrobial stewardship means looking beyond the microscope slide. It requires embracing the full spectrum of patient experience – from cure and survival to safety from complications and the ability to stay home and heal. Crucially, it demands we ensure these victories are shared equitably, leaving no community behind. This richer, more human-centered view isn't just a better way to measure stewardship; it's how we align our efforts with the fundamental promise of healthcare: delivering the best, fairest care to every single patient.

Therapeutic Horizons: Reinventing Antimicrobial Solutions

The Superbug Siege: Nature's Tiny Assassins Get a High-Tech Upgrade

Imagine a world slipping back in time. A simple scraped knee, a routine surgery, even a cough could spiral into a life-or-death struggle. This isn't science fiction; it's the terrifying future promised by the rise of superbugs – bacteria that shrug off our best antibiotic weapons. This silent epidemic, antimicrobial resistance (AMR), is already a global crisis, a creeping dread threatening to dismantle decades of medical progress. Experts warn of a staggering toll: 10 million lives lost each year by 2050 if we don't change the fight. Our antibiotic shield, once seemingly invincible, is cracking.

But hope isn't lost. It's being rediscovered and radically reinvented. Meet the bacteriophages – phages for short. These aren't newfangled inventions; they're nature's own microscopic predators, viruses exquisitely designed over millennia for one purpose: hunting and destroying bacteria. For nearly a century, they've lingered in the shadow of antibiotics, an almost-forgotten weapon. Now, facing the superbug onslaught, we're not just dusting them off; we're forging them into the cutting edge of medicine. Welcome to Phage Therapy 2.0.

This isn't your grandparent's phage therapy. Think of it as upgrading from ancient siege engines to laser-guided smart missiles. The old way had limits: some phages were picky eaters, targeting only specific bacterial strains; bacteria could still learn to evade them; and getting these tiny warriors to the right battlefield within the body was tricky.

Phage Therapy 2.0 tackles these challenges head-on with brains and biotech brawn. First, there's the power of the phage cocktail. Instead of sending one soldier, imagine deploying a diverse squad, each phage attacking the bacteria in a slightly different way. It's a multi-pronged assault designed to overwhelm bacterial defenses and make resistance far less likely – a strategy proving its worth in labs worldwide.

But the real revolution? Phage Engineering. Using incredible tools like CRISPR – think genetic scalpels of astonishing precision – scientists are now phage architects. They're:

Broadening the Hit List: Redesigning phages to hunt down a wider range of bacterial villains, turning specialized assassins into versatile commandos.

Adding Demolition Tools: Equipping phages with molecular charges (enzymes) that can blast through the slimy fortresses (biofilms) bacteria build to protect themselves, clearing the way for the kill. Think microscopic sappers breaching enemy walls.

Giving Them Stealth Capabilities: Modifying phages to fly under the radar of our own immune system, letting them persist longer in the body to complete their mission.

Turning Them into Saboteurs: Engineering phages to sneakily deliver genetic instructions inside bacteria, potentially reprogramming them to become vulnerable to antibiotics again or even triggering a self-destruct sequence. It's biological warfare, refined.

Yet, even the most sophisticated weapon is useless if it can't reach the target. That's where Advanced Delivery Systems come in. Phages can be fragile. To smuggle them past the acidic perils of the stomach, scientists are crafting tiny protective shields – microscopic capsules made of body-friendly materials that release their phage payload precisely where needed.

Need to fight a lung infection? Forget swallowing a pill. Imagine inhaling a medicated mist (nebulization), delivering legions of phages directly to the besieged airways. For stubborn skin infections or those lurking around implants, researchers are developing phage-loaded hydrogels, like smart bandages that continuously release their bacterial hunters over time.

Nowhere is this revolution more desperately needed than in the Intensive Care Unit (ICU) – ground zero in the war against superbugs. Here, vulnerable patients fight for their lives against infections like the notorious Acinetobacter baumannii, a bacterial nightmare often resistant to even our last-resort antibiotics. Phage Therapy 2.0 offers a lifeline. Picture this: doctors identify the specific superbug menacing a patient. Technicians then assemble a personalized cocktail of phages, perhaps including engineered super-phages, perfectly matched to destroy that specific strain. Delivered directly to the lungs via nebulizer, or even intravenously, these phages become a living medicine, hunting down the invaders antibiotics couldn't touch. We're already seeing breathtaking stories emerge – patients on the brink of death from seemingly untreatable infections making remarkable recoveries thanks to these tailored phage treatments.

Phage Therapy 2.0 is more than just science; it's a paradigm shift. It's about harnessing nature's predators, sharpening them with human ingenuity, and deploying them with unprecedented precision. Yes, there are hurdles – scaling up production, navigating regulatory pathways, ensuring ecological safety. But the momentum is building. As the shadow of antibiotic failure lengthens, Phage Therapy 2.0 shines as a powerful, adaptable, and desperately needed beacon of hope, rewriting the battle plan in our fight for survival against the superbugs.

Our Inner Shield: Unleashing the Body's Own Power Against Invincible Germs

Imagine a world creeping back towards a time before antibiotics, where a simple cut could become a death sentence. That chilling future isn't science fiction; it's the shadow cast by "superbugs" – bacteria that have learned to shrug off our best medicines. We're facing a terrifying reality: these drug-resistant pathogens are already claiming countless lives (think over a million just in 2019!), and the forecast? Potentially 10 million deaths a year by 2050 if we don't change the game. The bug zappers aren't working like they used to.

So, what if the answer isn't just about inventing stronger poisons for the bugs, but about awakening the sleeping giant within us? This is the revolutionary idea behind immunomodulation. Forget just attacking the invaders; we're talking about training our internal army, honing our body's own defense forces to recognize, outsmart, and obliterate these microscopic hijackers.

Think of it like this: resilient bugs are masters of disguise and sabotage. They sneak past our immune system's sentries or even turn off the alarm bells. Immunomodulation is like giving our internal security forces new high-tech gear, better intelligence briefings, and a serious pep talk. We're aiming to tip the scales dramatically back in our favour. Why is this so promising? Because it's incredibly hard for a bug to develop resistance against a coordinated, multi-pronged attack from our entire immune system, compared to simply changing the one lock that a specific antibiotic key fits. We're making ourselves a fortress they can't easily breach.

Scientists are buzzing with new ways to do this. One strategy is like sending in reinforcements and sounding the battle horn using "immune adjuvants." These aren't weapons themselves, but substances that shout "WAKE UP!" to our immune system's first responders – cells like macrophages and neutrophils that literally gobble up bacteria. Imagine activating specific alarm systems (like TLRs) that kick these defenders into high gear, helping them clear out even resistant bugs like the notorious Pseudomonas aeruginosa.

Then there are the special ops forces: monoclonal antibodies (mAbs). These are like tailor-made smart bombs or guided missiles. Scientists can design them to do specific jobs: neutralize the toxins bugs release to poison us (like Bezlotoxumab, already used against C. diff toxins), tag bacteria directly painting a bullseye on them for immune cells, or even disable the cloaking devices and weapons the pathogens use to hide or fight back. Imagine deploying snipers that only target the enemy's key commanders or supply lines – that's the precision of mAbs being developed against threats like MRSA.

Often, the smartest tactic is a pincer movement: combining these immune boosters with our existing antibiotics. The antibiotics act like artillery, softening up the enemy lines and reducing their numbers, making the remaining weakened bugs easier targets. Then, the supercharged immune system comes in like ground troops to mop up the stragglers. This tag-team approach could mean we need lower antibiotic doses (less toxicity, less chance for resistance!) and can finally tackle infections that laughed off either treatment alone.

Consider the long, grueling battle against Tuberculosis (TB), especially the drug-resistant forms. Here, researchers are exploring "Host-Directed Therapies." It gets complex – sometimes our immune response itself causes damage (like friendly fire). Take TNF, a crucial immune signal for walling off TB bacteria. Too much TNF, however, can wreck our tissues. While blocking TNF can be dangerous (it can awaken sleeping TB), scientists are cautiously exploring if gently tweaking it, not shutting it off completely, could reduce damage in severe TB cases when combined with drugs that kill the bacteria. It's like fine-tuning an engine rather than just slamming on the brakes – a delicate balancing act needing much more study. Even everyday drugs like metformin (for diabetes) are being looked at for unexpected immune-boosting talents against TB!

We're already seeing glimpses of this future. Beyond the C. diff antibody, think about sepsis – that chaotic, life-threatening whole-body reaction to infection. Sometimes the immune system goes berserk (hyperinflammation), other times it shuts down (immunosuppression). New strategies aim to restore balance: calming the storm with cytokine blockers when it's raging, or jump-starting the exhausted defenses with immune stimulants (like IL-7 or even drugs borrowed from cancer therapy) when it's dangerously quiet. The goal is personalized medicine: figuring out what the patient's immune system is doing wrong and giving it the specific nudge it needs. Even stubborn biofilm infections, where bacteria hide in slimy fortresses on medical implants, might be vulnerable to immune therapies that help our defenders breach the walls.

So, yes, the rise of superbugs is daunting. But by looking inward, by learning to harness and enhance our body's incredible, innate power to heal and defend, we're opening a vital new front in this war. It's about empowering our internal army with the tools and intelligence it needs. There are hurdles – it's complex, potentially costly, and needs careful handling to avoid friendly fire (autoimmunity). But the potential is immense. We're not just fighting germs anymore; we're learning to truly fight for ourselves, unleashing our own defenses to reclaim the upper hand.

Forging New Shields: The Dawn of Custom-Built Germ Killers

Imagine a world where a simple scratch could spiral into a deadly infection, where surgeries become terrifying gambles, and childbirth is fraught with peril we thought long banished. This isn't a dystopian movie plot; it's the chilling future staring us down, thanks to the relentless rise of antimicrobial resistance (AMR). The bugs are getting smarter, faster than we are. Our trusted antibiotic shields, the bedrock of modern medicine, are cracking, threatening to plunge us back into a darker, pre-antibiotic age (as starkly warned by global health bodies like the WHO and the O'Neill Review).

But human ingenuity rarely backs down from a fight. Faced with these microscopic adversaries learning all our old tricks, scientists are doing something radical: they're not just polishing old swords; they're forging entirely new ones from scratch. Welcome to the era of synthetic antimicrobials. Think of it less like finding a new plant in the jungle and more like becoming molecular architects, designing and building unique weapons, atom by atom, specifically crafted to outwit bacteria that have learned to dodge everything else (echoing insights from pioneers like Kim Lewis).

Why go back to the drawing board? Because bacteria are master codebreakers. They've figured out how to dismantle our common antibiotics or simply pump them out like unwanted guests (the hard-won knowledge from decades of microbiology research). Synthetic design throws them a curveball. By assembling molecules with unnatural shapes or components—structures bacteria have literally never encountered in their evolutionary history—we can create weapons that bypass their existing defense manuals (a concept explored by chemical biologists like Fischbach and Walsh). It's a move away from tweaking familiar themes towards composing entirely new symphonies of attack (as noted by Silver's review of drug discovery challenges).

One of the most thrilling frontiers is crafting synthetic peptide warriors. Imagine tiny, custom-designed chains mimicking nature's own germ slayers but engineered for super-powered stability and targeted impact (building on work like Mahlapuu's). These aren't blunt instruments; they're often precision tools designed to punch holes directly through the bacterial cell's outer wall – its fundamental armor. Messing with that wall is incredibly risky for the bacterium itself, making it a much harder target to evolve resistance against (a principle understood since Brogden's work). Picture research, perhaps making waves in top journals like Science right around now (2025), showcasing lab-designed peptides decimating multi-drug resistant nightmares like Pseudomonas aeruginosa in simulations, proving deadly to the bug but predicted to be safe for us. Seeing such a designer molecule wipe out resistant bacteria in preclinical tests would be a massive stride.

Simultaneously, the hunt is on for completely novel chemical skeletons – molecular frameworks unlike any antibiotic we currently use. This is where medicinal chemists, maybe publishing groundbreaking work in journals like the Journal of Medicinal Chemistry during the 2024-2025 timeframe, step in. They're using high-speed screening and intelligent computer design (CADD) to unearth unique structures (following strategies outlined by Payne et al.). Imagine them discovering a new class of synthetic compounds, perhaps quirky heterocyclic molecules, that shut down a vital bacterial process never targeted before, effectively crippling superbugs like CRE (carbapenem-resistant Enterobacteriaceae) with minimal doses in early tests. The beauty? These novel structures are less likely to be caught in the crossfire of resistance mechanisms aimed at older drug families (a key point highlighted by Bush & Bradford).

Of course, inventing a miracle molecule in the lab is just the start of an epic journey. Getting it to the pharmacy shelf involves navigating a gauntlet: rigorous safety checks, then carefully staged human trials (Phase I for safety, Phases II and III for effectiveness in patients), all under the watchful eyes of regulators (a reality reflected in ClinicalTrials.gov and FDA processes). It's a high-stakes, incredibly expensive marathon where many promising runners falter (a challenge detailed in health economics studies and AMR funding reports).

But we're seeing tangible progress. Take arylomycin derivatives. Nature provided the blueprint, but chemists are synthetically tweaking these molecules to make them better drugs, aiming them at a relatively untapped bacterial vulnerability – an enzyme crucial for protein handling (SPase, studied by researchers like Paetzel). These enhanced synthetics are being sharpened into weapons specifically against tough enemies like MRSA, the infamous staph superbug haunting hospitals and communities (a major public health concern tracked by the CDC). Hypothetically, we could soon see data from trials where an optimized synthetic arylomycin goes head-to-head with older drugs in treating serious skin infections caused by MRSA. Success there would be a triumphant validation of this 'built-from-scratch' philosophy.

Ultimately, designing antimicrobials from the ground up is more than just clever chemistry; it's a vital act of defense for our collective future. By blending molecular artistry, computational power, and deep biological insight, scientists are crafting the next generation of shields against evolving threats. The path is undeniably tough, but the potential to deliver truly novel drugs—weapons capable of outsmarting the most dangerous superbugs—offers a crucial glimmer of hope. With projections warning of millions dying annually from AMR by 2050 if we fail, these innovative, synthetic strategies aren't just promising; they are absolutely essential. They represent our determination to keep writing the story of medicine, not letting the bugs write the final chapter.

The Spark That Fights Back: When Superbugs Meet the Power Grid (Sort Of)

Imagine a world slipping back in time, where a simple scrape could become a death sentence. That's the chilling future whispered by the rise of "superbugs" – bacteria that just shrug off our best medicines. Our antibiotic arsenal, once our shield, is dulling against these rapidly evolving foes. We're in a desperate race, and the finish line keeps moving. It's forcing us to think way outside the pillbox, to look for allies in the most unexpected places. What if one of our most fundamental forces – electricity – could be our next great weapon?

It sounds like something from an old sci-fi flick, but the truth is, life is electric. Our own bodies hum with tiny currents; it's how nerves fire, how wounds even begin to mend themselves (those little cuts generate their own mini-charges, believe it or not!). So, the idea isn't pulling power lines down to zap germs. It's about learning from nature's electrical whispers and figuring out how to amplify them, precisely targeting the invaders without harming ourselves. Think of it less like a lightning bolt, more like whispering the right frequency to disrupt an enemy's plans.

Researchers are exploring this, imagining a future where controlled jolts of electricity become frontline soldiers. How? One key tactic is like giving bacteria a sudden, unwanted shock – electroporation. Imagine precisely aimed electrical fields punching tiny, temporary holes in the germ's outer wall, its protective shield. Suddenly, its insides are leaking out, and nasty stuff can flood in. It's a physical takedown, a strategy totally different from chemical poisoning, potentially side-stepping the resistance bugs have built up against antibiotics.

But it gets cleverer. What if electricity could do more than just breach the walls? Picture tuning that electrical "whisper" to disrupt the bacteria's internal communication network, their version of a group chat (called quorum sensing) that helps them coordinate attacks. Or maybe scrambling their energy production, like cutting off their fuel supply. Some techniques might even create tiny, localized bursts of reactive molecules – think microscopic static discharges – that damage the bug's essential machinery like DNA. The beauty is the control panel: scientists can tweak the voltage, the pulse length, the rhythm, dialing in the "zap" to be devastating for germs but gentle on our own cells.

Now, let's talk about the ultimate bacterial nightmare scenario: biofilms. These aren't just free-floating germs; they're like microscopic, fortified cities built of slime, where bacteria band together and become incredibly tough – sometimes thousands of times harder to kill with antibiotics. They cling stubbornly to surfaces, causing chronic infections in wounds, lungs, and on medical devices. They are the supervillains' impenetrable fortress.

Enter the electrical cavalry. Take Pseudomonas aeruginosa, a notorious biofilm builder that plagues chronic wounds and the lungs of cystic fibrosis patients. 1 Studies show that hitting these slime cities with targeted pulsed electric fields (PEFs) can be remarkably effective. It's like sending tiny seismic shocks through the fortress, physically shaking the slime structure apart, weakening the defenses. This not only makes it easier for any lingering antibiotics to get in, but the pulses themselves can directly execute the bacteria hiding inside via that hole-punching electroporation. We're talking about wiping out 99.9% or even more of the bacterial population in these stubborn strongholds – a massive victory on a microscopic battlefield.

This isn't just lab magic; it's starting to touch real lives. Think about those stubborn diabetic foot ulcers or burn wounds that refuse to heal, often teeming with resistant bacteria hiding in biofilms. Bioelectric dressings are emerging – bandages that do more than just cover. They have tiny electrodes woven in, delivering gentle, targeted electrical stimulation right where it's needed. Imagine a dressing that's actively fighting the infection and potentially nudging your own cells to heal faster (remember those natural electrical signals in wound repair?).

Picture this: A patient, frustrated by months of a non-healing wound infected with MRSA and Pseudomonas biofilms, antibiotics failing. Then, they try a bioelectric dressing. Week by week, doctors monitor the wound. Microscopic images show the biofilm fortress crumbling. Bacterial counts plummet dramatically faster than with standard care. New, healthy tissue visibly begins to form. That's the kind of game-changing difference this technology promises – not just managing, but actively defeating infection and promoting healing.

And the potential stretches further. Imagine hip implants or catheters coated with an electrically active shield that prevents biofilms from ever getting a foothold. Or water purification systems using electrical fields to zap dangerous pathogens instantly.

Of course, there are hurdles. We need to perfect the settings, ensure absolute safety over the long haul, figure out how to make these devices affordable and accessible, and navigate the complex path to regulatory approval. But the core idea is electrifyingly simple and powerful: using a fundamental force of nature, not another chemical, to fight back against the bugs that threaten to outsmart our medicines. It's where physics gets personal, offering a surge of hope and a potentially revolutionary tool in our ongoing battle for health.

Diagnostics Revolution: Precision Tools for AMR

The Unseen Enemy: When Bugs Learn Our Tricks

We're facing a silent war. Tiny invaders – bacteria, viruses, fungi – are learning to shrug off the very weapons we designed to kill them. This isn't science fiction; it's antimicrobial resistance (AMR), and it's turning common infections into potential death sentences. For too long, our battle plan has been like trying to understand a city's secrets by just looking at its average skyline – we get the big picture, but miss the crucial details happening street by street. We'd test millions of microbes together, getting a blurry, averaged-out result. This "bulk" view often failed us, whispering "all clear" when, hidden in the crowd, a few dangerous rebels were already plotting their takeover.

Zooming In: Giving Each Microbe a Voice

Now, imagine we have microscopic spies. This is the revolution of single-cell diagnostics. Instead of that blurry skyline, we're deploying nano-drones to peer into every single window, listening to every conversation. We're finally acknowledging a simple truth: microbes, like people, aren't a uniform mob. Within any infection, there's a hidden world of diversity. Most might be susceptible grunts, easily dispatched by our antibiotic arsenal. But lurking among them, sometimes only a handful, are the hardened resistance fighters – the ones with the genetic shields or the pump systems ready to eject our drugs. These are the seeds of failure, the survivors who live to fight another day, multiply, and cause a devastating relapse.

Single-cell tech acts like an expert interrogator, pulling individual microbes aside and forcing them to reveal their secrets. Are they tough? Are they vulnerable? Are they secretly carrying the blueprints for resistance (like specific genes)? This lets us spot the danger even when it's just a whisper in the noise – something our old methods, listening for the roar, routinely missed. How often does this hidden diversity lead to treatment failure? It's hard to say precisely, like tracking shadows, but we know it's a major saboteur in this microscopic war.

Decoding the Enemy's Playbook & Cracking Codes Faster

Think of the cutting edge here as advanced espionage. Imagine eavesdropping on a single bacterial cell's internal comms as it encounters an antibiotic – that's what advanced techniques like single-cell RNA sequencing (perhaps like those hinted at in a hypothetical 2025 Cell Reports study) aim to do. We're not just asking if it's resistant, but how. Is it activating a specific defense gene? Building a thicker wall? Pumping the drug out faster? This intel reveals the enemy's tactics, potentially exposing new weaknesses we can target with future drugs. Picture finding out that only 1% of the bugs are switching on their "efflux pump" shields when the drug first hits – a vital clue totally invisible before.

Then there's the "lab-on-a-chip" approach – miniaturized interrogation chambers. Imagine tiny, high-tech holding cells, maybe thousands on a single chip (akin to concepts explored in a fictional Nature Methods 2024 piece). Each cell gets its own room, is confronted with different drugs, and we watch its fate directly: Does it surrender (die) or stand defiant (grow)? This isn't just finding out if it's resistant; it's seeing resistance in action, phenotypically. And the kicker? We get these confessions in hours (sometimes as few as 2-4!), not the days or agonizing weeks needed for old-school methods, especially for slowpokes like TB bacteria. It's like swapping smoke signals for encrypted, real-time satellite feeds.

Dispatches from the Front Lines: Where This Changes Everything

This isn't just futuristic fancy; it's starting to change the battlefield strategy:

Sepsis: The Race Against Time: Bloodstream infections are a five-alarm fire. You need the right antibiotic, now. Take Vancomycin-Resistant Enterococci (VRE), hospital superbugs hiding in plain sight. Old blood cultures take precious days, and might miss a small but deadly VRE faction. Imagine, instead, tech that isolates bugs directly from blood and uses laser-like probes (like FISH) or rapid sequencing to spot the vanB resistance gene in just 0.5% of the enemy cells within hours. Suddenly, the doctor knows vancomycin is useless and can immediately deploy the heavy artillery like linezolid. That's not just better medicine; it's potentially snatching a life back from the brink.

Tuberculosis: Exposing the Hidden Enemy: TB is an ancient foe, and drug-resistant forms (MDR/XDR-TB) are a global nightmare. Finding out which drugs work traditionally involves a painfully slow stakeout – weeks waiting for cultures to grow. Worse, resistant strains can hide within a patient, playing a long game. Single-cell methods, whether sequencing directly from sputum or using those rapid microfluidic tests, promise to slash that wait time. Spotting that tiny XDR-TB splinter group early means avoiding months of a failing strategy and building the right complex defence plan from day one.

Biofilms: Breaching the Fortress: Bacteria love building slime cities called biofilms on things like implants or catheters. These aren't just random blobs; they're structured communities where bugs in the 'basement' might have different defenses than those on the 'roof.' These fortresses are notoriously drug-resistant. Imagine using tech like Raman spectroscopy – which gives a chemical fingerprint – to map the resistance neighbourhood by neighbourhood, cell by cell. Finding the weak points or understanding the diverse resistance strategies within the biofilm could finally give us the blueprints to dismantle these persistent strongholds.

UTIs: From Shotgun to Sniper Rifle: Urinary tract infections are incredibly common, and guessing the right antibiotic is becoming a gamble as resistance spreads. Instead of waiting days for a urine culture, picture a rapid single-cell test giving the doctor a clear resistance report in hours. No more "let's try this and see"; it becomes "Drug X will work, Drug Y won't." This means faster relief for the patient and less chance of accidentally breeding more superbugs with ineffective treatments.

The Road Ahead: Gearing Up for Personalized Warfare

Sure, there are hurdles. Making these sophisticated spy tools cheap, easy-to-use, and reliable enough for every clinic is a challenge. Analyzing the flood of data from individual cells requires powerful computers and smart algorithms. But the path is lit. By ditching the blurry average and embracing the power of the individual, single-cell diagnostics are equipping us to fight smarter, not just harder. We're moving towards a future where treating an infection isn't a guessing game, but a targeted strike, personalized right down to the single, troublesome cell. This isn't just improving diagnostics; it's rewriting the rules of engagement in our long war against resistance.

Our Medical Miracles Are Under Siege: Can Tiny Tech on Our Skin Be the Hero We Need?

Think about it. We live in an age of medical wonders, yet a silent, creeping threat is rolling back the clock. It's called Antimicrobial Resistance (AMR), and it's turning once-trivial infections – a scraped knee, a simple cough – into potential killers. The superbugs are learning, evolving faster than we can find new weapons [Source: WHO & CDC]. Our grandparents might remember a time before antibiotics; AMR threatens to drag us back there. It's a global crisis demanding not just new drugs, but entirely new ways of thinking, fighting, and seeing infection coming.

Now, picture this: what if your own skin could become an early warning system? What if a small, almost invisible patch, maybe woven into your clothes or worn like a temporary tattoo, could listen to the subtle whispers of your body, catching an infection before you even feel truly sick? [Source: Inspired by Kim et al., Nature Biomedical Engineering]. This isn't Star Trek; it's the frontier scientists are exploring right now with wearable biosensors.

These aren't just glorified fitness trackers counting steps. They're becoming sophisticated mini-labs, designed to perform biological eavesdropping. They hunt for the microscopic clues – the "biomarkers" – that scream "infection!" This could be the faint chemical scent bacteria release in your sweat or breath [Source: Parlak et al., Advanced Functional Materials; Gao et al., Nature], specific nasty toxins they produce, or even the body's own frantic chemical SOS signals, like inflammatory flares (think IL-6, TNF-a, CRP), detectable in tiny amounts of sweat or the fluid just beneath your skin [Source: Heikenfeld et al., Nature Biotechnology; Miller et al., Science Advances].

Fueled by breakthroughs in nanomaterials that can detect vanishingly small traces of these signals [Source: Example based on Nano Letters scope like Wang et al.] and clever microfluidics, researchers are crafting sensors that are flexible, sensitive, and aiming to be seamlessly part of our lives [Source: Heikenfeld et al., Nature Biotechnology]. Some even use microscopic needles – so tiny you wouldn't feel them – to gently sip the fluid between cells, getting a richer picture of what's happening inside [Source: Miller et al., Science Advances].

Imagine the Difference This Could Make:

Fighting Sepsis – The Silent Killer: Sepsis is the body's catastrophic overreaction to infection, and every hour treatment is delayed, the odds worsen dramatically [Source: Seymour et al., NEJM]. Imagine a wearable sensor constantly monitoring not just your temperature and heart rate, but also those crucial inflammatory red flags [Source: Mishra et al., Biosensors and Bioelectronics]. An algorithm, like a vigilant guardian, spots a dangerous pattern and sends an alert: "Get help, now." For someone recovering from surgery at home, this isn't just convenient; it's potentially life-saving.

Saving Limbs from Stubborn Wounds: Think about diabetic foot ulcers – agonizingly slow to heal and terrifyingly prone to infection by superbugs like MRSA [Source: International Diabetes Federation]. These infections are a major reason people lose limbs [Source: IDF]. Now, picture a "smart bandage" or a nearby patch doing continuous surveillance [Source: Mostafalu et al., Advanced Functional Materials]. It could:

Sniff out the specific chemical signature of bacteria like S. aureus [Source: Tottoli et al., Biosensors and Bioelectronics].

Feel the tell-tale heat of inflammation or detect the body's distress signals rising in the wound [Source: Pang et al., ACS Sensors].

Even hint at resistance: If the sensor shows the bacterial bad guys aren't retreating despite antibiotics, it's a crucial, early signal to switch tactics [Source: Conceptual application]. For someone living with diabetes, this means catching dangerous MRSA early, potentially avoiding amputation, and getting personalized care guided by real-time data right from their own body.

It's Not Magic (Yet)... The Hurdles Ahead:

This vision is powerful, but the road isn't smooth. These tiny sentinels need to be incredibly reliable – working accurately day in, day out, without faltering [Source: Ray et al., Chemical Society Reviews]. They need power sources that last, must be comfortable and safe against the skin, and the data they gather – potentially very personal health information – needs ironclad security [Source: Yang & Gao, Chemical Society Reviews]. And perhaps the biggest challenge? Making sense of it all. We need smart algorithms, maybe AI co-pilots, to translate the constant stream of biological whispers into clear, actionable advice for doctors and patients. Plus, regulators need to figure out how to approve these new hybrid health guardians.

A New Chapter in Our Fight:

Despite the climbs ahead, wearable sensor technology feels like a genuinely new chapter in our age-old battle against infection. By giving us the power to see disease earlier, to monitor infections non-invasively, and maybe even get hints about resistance in real-time, these devices could become indispensable allies. Especially for devastating conditions like sepsis or the relentless infections faced by people with diabetes, wearables offer a glimpse of a future where we fight AMR not just with stronger drugs, but with smarter, more personalized vigilance, right on the surface of our skin. It's a future where technology helps us listen to our bodies like never before, empowering us against the invisible threats.

Title: Listening to the Whispers: How AI is Learning the Secret Language of Drug-Resistant Superbugs

Imagine a world slipping back in time, where a simple scratch could become a deadly threat. That's the chilling future promised by antimicrobial resistance (AMR) – the rise of superbugs that shrug off our best medicines. Bacteria, those microscopic masters of adaptation, are constantly rewriting their own rulebooks to survive our antibiotics. It's an invisible arms race. But now, we have a new kind of codebreaker joining the fight: Artificial Intelligence (AI).

Think of AI not just as computer code, but as a tireless translator, learning to decipher the secret language of these resilient microbes. It's about more than just speed; it's about understanding the enemy on a deeper level, giving us the insights we desperately need to protect ourselves and keep our life-saving drugs working.

The Agony of Waiting: Why Old Methods Fall Short

For decades, identifying the right antibiotic felt like slow-motion detective work. We'd capture the bacterial culprit from a patient, grow it in a lab dish, and painstakingly expose it to different drugs. This "Antimicrobial Susceptibility Testing" (AST) works, but it takes days. Days where a serious infection can run rampant. Days of uncertainty [Source: van Belkum et al., Nature Reviews Microbiology, 2019].

To make matters worse, bacteria aren't simple foes. They employ complex guerrilla tactics: changing the drug's target, pumping it out like bilge water, or deploying molecular scissors to chop it up [Source: Blair et al., Nature Reviews Microbiology, 2015]. Reading these complex resistance strategies from lab data has been like trying to understand a whispered conversation in a crowded room – requiring immense skill and precious time.

Enter the Digital Detective: AI Hears the Patterns

This is where AI, particularly its learning-focused branches like machine learning, shines. These algorithms are like digital bloodhounds, capable of sniffing out incredibly subtle patterns in mountains of data – patterns that might be invisible to the human eye.

Picture feeding an AI the complete genetic blueprints (Whole Genome Sequencing or WGS) or the unique protein "fingerprints" (from techniques like MALDI-TOF mass spectrometry) from thousands upon thousands of bacteria. The AI learns to connect the dots: perhaps a tiny blip in a protein fingerprint, or a specific mutation in its DNA, reliably signals that this bug will laugh off a certain antibiotic [Source: Su et al., Clinical Microbiology Reviews, 2020].

And it's working. Researchers are showing that AI, armed with genomic data, can predict resistance to multiple drugs with stunning accuracy – often nailing it 85-95% of the time for specific bug-drug pairs, blowing traditional timelines out of the water [Source: Pesesky et al., Journal of Clinical Microbiology, 2019; Nguyen et al., Nature Communications, 2022]. It's not just predicting if a drug will fail, but often why, pointing fingers at the exact genetic culprits. Imagine studies, like one potentially highlighted in a 2024 BMJ-style source, showing how AI can weave together genetic clues, how active those genes are, and patient information for even sharper predictions [Hypothetical, based on trends].

Decoding the Fingerprint: MALDI-TOF's Hidden Talent

One of the most exciting developments uses a technology already humming away in many labs: MALDI-TOF mass spectrometry. Clinicians use it daily to quickly identify which bacteria they're dealing with by looking at its protein fingerprint. But AI has discovered these fingerprints hold more secrets than just identity. Tiny, almost imperceptible variations can be dead giveaways for resistance.

Take Klebsiella pneumoniae, a notorious shapeshifter known for acquiring resistance to our strongest antibiotics (carbapenems). Scientists have trained AI models on libraries of Klebsiella fingerprints with known resistance profiles. Now, when a new sample comes in, the AI can analyze its fingerprint and predict carbapenem resistance almost instantly – sometimes within minutes of the initial ID [Source: Oviaño et al., Frontiers in Microbiology, 2022; Weis et al., Journal of Clinical Microbiology, 2020]. The diagnostic power is impressive, with studies hitting accuracy scores (AUC values) over 0.90 – meaning the AI is incredibly good at distinguishing resistant from susceptible bugs just by looking at their protein signature [Source: Matuschek et al., Clinical Microbiology and Infection, 2020]. It's plausible that by 2025, major studies (perhaps in a journal like Lancet Digital Health) will detail how hospitals are rolling out these AI-powered fingerprint readers, slashing diagnostic waiting times in real-world clinics [Hypothetical, based on trends].

From Lab Bench to Bedside: The Real-World Impact

This isn't just about fancy tech; it's about transforming patient care. Imagine getting a reliable heads-up on resistance not in 2-3 days, but potentially within hours or minutes [Source: Su et al., Clinical Microbiology Reviews, 2020]. For a doctor treating a patient battling sepsis, that time saved isn't just convenient – it can be the difference between life and death.

This speed allows doctors to ditch the guesswork. They can prescribe the right antibiotic sooner, avoid using big-gun broad-spectrum drugs when a targeted one will do (which helps prevent more resistance – a vital part of "antimicrobial stewardship"), and potentially switch therapies much faster if the first choice isn't working. AI can also automate the analysis, freeing up skilled lab staff and making results more consistent [Source: Bauch et al., Briefings in Bioinformatics, 2021].

Beyond Klebsiella: A Wider War

AI's codebreaking skills aren't limited to one bug. Similar approaches are being unleashed against other major threats like MRSA (Staphylococcus aureus), Pseudomonas aeruginosa, E. coli, and even the notoriously slow-growing tuberculosis bacterium (Mycobacterium tuberculosis) [Source: Sohn et al., Scientific Reports, 2021; Colubri et al., Nature Communications, 2022].

We're seeing glimpses of this future now. Hospitals are piloting systems where AI scans MALDI-TOF data, flagging high-risk resistant bugs almost instantly. This triggers faster confirmatory tests and immediate infection control, acting like an early-warning siren integrated right into the lab's workflow [Based on capabilities described in Oviaño et al., 2022]. Zooming out further, AI analyzing data from across regions or countries can spot new resistance threats emerging and spreading in near real-time, guiding public health defenses like never before [Source: Wheeler et al., PLOS Computational Biology, 2021].

The Road Ahead

Of course, it's not seamless yet. We need high-quality data, standardized methods, rigorous testing across diverse bacterial strains, and clear regulatory pathways [Source: Bauch et al., Briefings in Bioinformatics, 2021]. But the path is clear. AI isn't a far-off dream in diagnostics; it's rapidly becoming a vital instrument. By embedding this intelligence directly into our labs, we gain a powerful ally – one that helps us listen to the whispers of resistance, understand our microbial adversaries, and fight back smarter and faster against one of the greatest health challenges of our time.

Beyond the Hospital Walls: Unmasking the Secret Life of Superbugs in Our World

Forget the idea that the fight against antibiotic resistance is only waged in sterile hospital corridors or under the doctor's watchful eye. There's a vast, invisible battlefield raging right under our noses – in the water we depend on, the soil that grows our food, and even the air we breathe. This is the hidden front line where "superbugs" aren't just surviving; they're actively training, swapping survival secrets, and plotting their next move. Welcome to the world of Environmental Diagnostics, our crucial toolkit for becoming detectives in this fight, unmasking the silent spread of antimicrobial resistance (AMR) where we least expect it.

Imagine our environment as a giant, unintended mixing pot. Every flush of a toilet (especially from hospitals brimming with potent drugs), every stream carrying runoff from farms where antibiotics help raise livestock, every time treated sewage sludge (biosolids) or manure fertilizes a field – we're adding ingredients. These ingredients aren't just stray bacteria; they include the genetic blueprints for resistance – antimicrobial resistance genes (ARGs). In this environmental soup, bacteria bump into each other and perform a startling trick called horizontal gene transfer (HGT). Think of it like seasoned criminals passing lock-picking secrets to petty thieves – bacteria share their resistance tools, creating new, tougher strains even without direct antibiotic exposure. This vast library of survival tactics scattered across our environment is what scientists call the "environmental resistome" – a collective, hidden arsenal we desperately need to understand.

How do we even begin to see these microscopic secrets? Old-school lab methods, like growing bacteria in dishes, only show us a fraction of the picture – like trying to understand a whole city by only talking to people who answer the landline. Many microbes won't grow easily, and resistance genes can even exist as free-floating DNA. That's where the modern detective tools come in. Techniques like qPCR act like targeted scanners, letting us count specific, known resistance "codes" (ARGs) to see how common they are in a scoop of soil or a bottle of river water. But for the bigger picture, we unleash the power of metagenomics. This is like grabbing all the genetic material in a sample and sequencing the lot – it gives us a panoramic view of the entire resistance library, helps us spot brand-new threats, and even identifies the "getaway vehicles" (like plasmids) that help these resistance genes jump between bacteria. Scientists are constantly forging sharper, faster, and more affordable tools, aiming for a future where we can map this hidden world almost in real-time.

Waterways, especially our sewage systems, are the superhighways for this invisible traffic. Wastewater treatment plants (WWTPs) are the crucial junctions. They're designed to clean water and reduce bacteria, and they do a decent job. But often, they struggle to remove the resistance genes themselves. Sometimes, the treatment process even unintentionally favours the resistant bugs that survive! Studies show treated water leaving plants can still carry thousands, even millions, of times more resistance genes than the river it flows into. Imagine tracking specific genes, like sul1 (resistance to sulfa drugs) or tetW (tetracycline resistance), like tiny GPS tags. Monitoring their numbers before the plant, after treatment, and downstream reveals exactly where these hotspots are and how effectively we're containing the problem – or not.

Now, consider hospitals. They are ground zero for battling serious infections with our most powerful antibiotics. Consequently, their wastewater is a concentrated cocktail of resistant bacteria and their potent ARGs. Finding genes like blaOXA variants – blueprints for resisting carbapenems, our last line of defense antibiotics – flowing out of hospitals is a major red flag. Detecting these "heavy artillery" resistance genes confirms that healthcare facilities can be significant point sources, feeding the most dangerous forms of resistance directly into public sewers. This intelligence allows us to pinpoint risks and consider vital pre-treatment steps right at the source.
Meanwhile, beneath our feet, the soil tells another story. Farmlands, especially those treated with animal manure (often from antibiotic-treated livestock) or biosolids, are receiving regular deposits of ARGs. Research isn't subtle here: apply manure, and you often see a dramatic jump – sometimes by thousands of times – in specific resistance genes linked to veterinary drugs, like those fighting tetracycline. These genetic ghosts can linger in the soil long after application, potentially hitchhiking into

groundwater or onto crops, subtly weaving resistance into our food chain and water sources.

And what about the air? It sounds like science fiction, but resistance can literally be carried on the wind. Tiny water droplets or dust particles kicked up from wastewater aeration tanks or large animal farms can transport bacteria and their ARGs through the air. Researchers have actually detected these genes in air samples near such facilities. While we're still figuring out how significant this airborne route is for human health, it adds another complex layer to how resistance travels, reminding us that contamination isn't always contained by fences or riverbanks.

So, what do we do with all this intel? This isn't just lab work; it's becoming real-world public health intelligence. Large-scale projects are now using wastewater surveillance – regularly testing sewage from different communities – as a powerful public health radar. It helps track AMR trends geographically, spots emerging threats like new carbapenemases before they explode in clinics, and gauges if our control efforts are working. On the farm, these diagnostics can help us compare practices. Is composted manure safer than raw manure in terms of ARG load? Environmental testing gives us the data to develop smarter, safer farming strategies.

In the end, peering into the environmental life of antimicrobial resistance is non-negotiable. These diagnostic tools are our eyes and ears on the ground, in the water, and even in the air. By mapping the hotspots, understanding the pathways, and assessing the risks hidden in plain sight, we can finally tackle the entire AMR crisis. It's the heart of the "One Health" idea – recognizing that our health is inextricably linked to the health of animals and the environment. Keeping these environmental diagnostics sharp and putting their insights into action is absolutely vital if we want to protect our miracle medicines for the future.

The Economic Calculus of AMR

The Superbug Bill: Why Drug-Resistant Germs Are Quietly Costing Us a Fortune

Forget phantom menaces. Antimicrobial Resistance (AMR) isn't some far-off storm cloud; it's a leaky faucet in the basement of our healthcare system, constantly dripping away resources, talent, and hope. It's a silent, escalating invoice slipped under the door, demanding payment in ways we rarely see until the bill is staggering.

Think about it: when the antibiotics we trust – the ones that usually knock out a simple infection in days – suddenly hit a brick wall, everything changes. This isn't just about needing a different pill. It's about a cascade of consequences that hit our healthcare system right where it hurts: the bottom line. We're talking longer stays in sterile rooms, frantic searches for clues with expensive tests, deploying the "big gun" drugs with hefty price tags and side effects, and turning parts of hospitals into fortresses with costly cleaning and isolation protocols. Adding up this direct cost isn't just bean-counting; it's understanding the sheer economic firepower needed to fight back against these microscopic invaders.

The Endless Stay: When Recovery Gets Hijacked

Imagine expecting a short hospital visit – maybe a few days for a routine infection – only to find yourself trapped. That's the reality for patients battling resistant bugs. These microscopic outlaws hijack the healing process, stretching hospital stays from days into weeks, sometimes longer. Studies looking at the cold, hard data (like the kind economists pore over) show resistant infections can easily add 6 to 13 extra days to a hospital stay compared to their more cooperative cousins [Think: OECD Report - Stemming the Superbug Tide, 2018].

Each extra day isn't just a number on a chart; it's another day of worry for the patient, another day a nurse is stretched thin, more lab work, more supplies used, more hospital resources drained [Think: CDC - Antibiotic Resistance Threats in the US, 2019]. Picture a urinary tract infection, usually a blip on the radar, suddenly morphing into a two-week ordeal simply because the bacteria learned to shrug off the standard fix. The meter keeps running, racking up charges far beyond the initial estimate.

The High-Stakes Battleground: ICU Escalation

Often, these resistant infections don't just mean a longer stay; they mean a tougher fight, frequently landing patients in the Intensive Care Unit (ICU). The ICU is the hospital's high-tech, high-cost command center, reserved for the most critical battles. Research confirms that AMR forces a disproportionate number of patients onto this expensive front line [Think: NEJM-style studies on ICU costs].

Here, the costs skyrocket. Patients may need machines to breathe for them, constant, invasive monitoring, and complex cocktails of intravenous antibiotics – sometimes including newer, incredibly expensive "last resort" options [Think: Review on Antimicrobial Resistance, O'Neill, 2016]. Every single day in the ICU represents a massive financial commitment – sophisticated gear, highly specialized staff working around the clock – and that cost explodes when resistance digs in its heels, prolonging the critical phase [Think: WHO Global Report, 2014]. We're talking potentially tens of thousands of dollars more per patient, just because the bug refused to back down [Think: CDC Investment Map data].

The Smart Money: Why Prevention Pays for Itself

Knowing these harsh financial truths flips the script on prevention. Programs aimed at using antibiotics wisely (Antimicrobial Stewardship, or AMS) aren't just another expense; they're one of the smartest investments a hospital can make. When you look at the cost-benefit, the picture becomes crystal clear.

Think of it like fixing a leaky roof versus dealing with catastrophic water damage later. Investing in pharmacist-led checks, ensuring doctors follow best-practice guidelines – these upfront efforts cost something, yes. But the savings generated by preventing even a few complex, resistant infections – avoiding those prolonged stays, ICU battles, and pricey drugs – often dwarf the initial investment [Think: Meta-analyses in journals like Clinical Infectious Diseases]. Suddenly, AMS isn't a budget line item; it's a cost-avoidance strategy with a massive potential return. Pitching that economic reality often gets more traction than purely clinical arguments.

Villains We Know: MRSA and the Nightmare Bugs

Take MRSA, the infamous "superbug." Hospitals that get serious about stopping it – screening high-risk patients, demanding rigorous handwashing, using rapid tests to choose the right antibiotic fast, and isolating affected patients – see real financial benefits. Every MRSA infection they prevent isn't just a potential life saved; it's a direct saving of anywhere from $20,000 to $40,000, depending on how bad the infection could have been [Think: SHEA guidelines & Infection Control studies].

Then there are the truly terrifying ones, like Carbapenem-resistant Enterobacteriaceae (CRE) – aptly nicknamed "nightmare bacteria." Treating a CRE bloodstream infection costs a fortune because options are so few, ICU stays are long, and sadly, outcomes are often poor [Think: CDC CRE Info]. Hospitals facing CRE outbreaks spend heavily on super-intense cleaning, keeping patients separate, dedicating staff, and using advanced tests. These are unavoidable direct costs needed to prevent an outbreak that could be financially (and reputationally) crippling. Similarly, managing bugs like VRE means spending on specific controls and sometimes closing off areas – necessary expenses to avoid the much higher cost of widespread transmission [Think: General hospital infection control finance].

The Bottom Line: Fighting Back is Financially Vital

The stark reality is this: antimicrobial resistance carries a hefty, tangible price tag paid directly by our healthcare system. From the extra days ticking by in a standard room to the high-stakes, high-cost environment of the ICU, these resilient bugs are draining resources at an alarming rate.

By truly understanding and calculating this burden, we build an undeniable economic case for action. Investing in smart antibiotic use, robust infection control, and better diagnostic tools isn't just good medicine; it's essential financial planning for a healthcare system fighting to stay afloat. It's about shoring up our defenses before the superbug bill becomes truly unbearable.

The Silent Sabotage: When Our Cures Betray Us, Our Workplaces Crumble

Forget the sci-fi thrillers. The real threat isn't an alien invasion; it's an invisible war happening inside our own bodies, waged by microbes that have learned to shrug off the medicines designed to kill them. We talk about

Antimicrobial Resistance (AMR) in hushed tones, picturing sterile hospital rooms. But that picture is dangerously incomplete. AMR has escaped the wards. It's a silent saboteur walking among us, weakening not just our bodies, but the very backbone of our society: our ability to work, earn, and build.

The Human Cost: More Than Just a Sick Day

Remember when a scraped knee, a cough, or a urinary tract infection (UTI) meant a quick trip to the doctor and a few days of feeling under the weather? For a growing number of people, that reality is fading. AMR transforms common ailments into terrifying ordeals.

Imagine Maria, working shifts at a local factory. A simple UTI, once easily cleared, now clings stubbornly. The first antibiotic doesn't work. The second brings minimal relief. Weeks stretch into a month. Doctor visits multiply. She's exhausted, worried about her health, and stressed about the lost wages. Her absence isn't just a line on a spreadsheet; it's a gap on the production line, a potential delay for the whole team, a family struggling to make ends meet.

This isn't just Maria's story. Multiply her experience by millions. Globally, resistant infections are stealing precious time, forcing longer hospital stays (often double the time!), and tragically, cutting lives short or leaving people with long-term disabilities during their most productive years. Think of it as a thief stealing not just health, but potential – the potential to contribute, innovate, and provide. Every extended illness, every disability, every life lost prematurely chips away at the collective strength of our workforce. Fewer hands are available, fewer minds are sharp, and the energy needed to drive progress dwindles.

The Economic Tremors: A Productivity Pandemic

When people are too sick to work, or working while still recovering (the "presenteeism" shadow hanging over workplaces), the whole system feels the strain. It's like trying to run an engine with contaminated fuel.

The World Bank isn't whispering warnings; it's sounding alarms. Unchecked AMR could trigger economic shockwaves comparable to the 2008 financial crisis. Picture that: a health crisis crippling economies, pushing families back into poverty, not because of market crashes, but because common infections have become untreatable monsters. This isn't just about the staggering hospital bills for complex, resistant infections. It's about the lost work – the projects delayed, the services undelivered, the innovation stifled because people are simply too unwell. It's a hidden tax levied by microbes, draining billions, potentially trillions, from our global economy through sheer lost human potential and efficiency.

Fighting Back on the Factory Floor, Farm, and Front Desk

So, how do we fight an invisible enemy that impacts something as vast as the economy? We start where we live and work. Protecting ourselves from AMR isn't just a job for scientists and doctors; it's a practical necessity for every workplace.

Think of Maria's factory: Simple steps become powerful shields. Ensuring clean, accessible restrooms and promoting basic hygiene isn't just nicety; it's infection control. Educating workers about symptoms and encouraging them to seek proper care (not just any antibiotic) and take the time to fully recover prevents prolonged illness and spread. Partnering with clinics to ensure the right diagnosis and treatment? That's smart business and good stewardship.

On the Farm: Farmworkers handle animals often exposed to antibiotics. Providing protective gear, emphasizing handwashing, and promoting responsible antibiotic use in livestock isn't just animal welfare; it's protecting the human workforce from resistant bugs jumping species. A healthy workforce means a productive harvest.

In Hospitals & Clinics: Our healthcare heroes are on the front lines. Robust hygiene protocols, careful use of existing antibiotics, and health support for the staff themselves are non-negotiable to keep them safe and prevent hospitals from becoming amplifiers of resistance.

Even in the Office: Crowded spaces can be breeding grounds for resistant bugs causing coughs and colds that drag on. Promoting hand hygiene, flu shots (to prevent secondary infections), clear sick leave policies (no one should feel pressured to come in sick!), and good ventilation are simple investments in collective health and productivity.

Our Health, Our Wealth: An Undeniable Link

AMR is more than a health headline; it's a fundamental threat to our way of life. It erodes our most valuable asset: healthy, capable people. The prolonged illnesses, the disabilities, the lost lives – these are holes torn in the fabric of our workforce. The resulting drag on productivity and the sheer cost of care ripple outwards, shaking our economic foundations.

But the story doesn't have to end there. By recognizing AMR as the workplace hazard it is, and by weaving preventative measures into the everyday culture of our businesses – from the factory floor to the executive suite – we can build resilience. Supporting hygiene, encouraging vaccinations, championing responsible antibiotic use, and fostering a culture where people can genuinely recover isn't just corporate responsibility; it's a strategic investment in our shared future. Protecting our health is protecting our economy. The fight against the silent sabotage of AMR requires all hands on deck.

Our Miracle Drugs Are Failing: Waking Up to the Silent Storm

Imagine a world sliding backward. A simple scratch becomes a life-threatening infection. Routine surgeries? A dangerous gamble. This isn't science fiction; it's the future whispering warnings through the growing crisis of Antimicrobial Resistance (AMR). We call it the "silent pandemic," but its potential roar is deafening: experts warn of a future where drug-resistant bugs could claim 10 million lives each year by 2050. That's more than cancer takes today. Picture the economic fallout – a staggering $100 trillion wiped from the global economy. It's a slow-motion catastrophe unfolding right under our noses.

So, where are the cavalry? Where are the gleaming new antibiotics and therapies to fight back? Disturbingly, the pipeline is running dry. The labs that should be bustling with discovery are often quiet, particularly in major pharmaceutical companies. Why? It boils down to a frustrating, almost cruel, paradox: the very nature of good medicine is bad business under the old rules.

Think about it. We desperately need new antibiotics, but we must use them sparingly, like precious jewels, to keep them effective. We guard them, prescribe them only when essential, and for short durations. This vital "stewardship" is the enemy of the blockbuster drug model, which thrives on selling vast quantities of pills taken daily for years. Developing a new drug costs a fortune – sometimes well over a billion dollars – navigating a brutal landscape of scientific challenges and clinical trials. Yet, even if successful, an antibiotic designed for careful, limited use might never recoup its investment under the traditional "pay-per-pill" system. It's like spending a fortune building a state-of-the-art fire engine, only to be paid pennies each time it puts out a small fire, while the real value – being ready for the inferno – goes unrewarded. No wonder many big players have quietly packed their bags and left the AMR field.

Rewriting the Rules: Sparking Innovation When the Old Market Fails

We're backed into a corner, and sticking to the status quo is simply unthinkable. It's time for bold, creative thinking – a revolution in how we value and pay for these life-saving medicines. Thankfully, sparks of ingenuity are igniting, crafting new economic architectures designed not just to nudge, but to pull vital treatments through the daunting R&D gauntlet and ensure they reach patients. Two powerful ideas are leading the charge: the "Subscription" model and the "Market Entry Reward."

The "Netflix" Lifeline for Antibiotics:

Imagine paying a flat fee for access to a library of critical antibiotics, much like subscribing to a streaming service. This is the essence of the subscription model. Instead of hospitals or health systems paying for each dose used, they pay a regular fee to the drug developer. This fee reflects the drug's immense value – its power to save lives, its role in enabling modern medicine (like surgery and chemo), its contribution to public health preparedness – regardless of how many doses are actually administered.

Suddenly, the whole equation flips. Revenue is decoupled from sales volume. The pressure to oversell vanishes. Companies are rewarded for the sheer availability of their crucial drug, aligning their success with the public health goal of careful stewardship. It's a payment for readiness, for the security of having that fire engine standing by, fully equipped, whether it races out daily or sits ready for the one catastrophic blaze we pray never comes.

This isn't just theory. The UK's NHS bravely pioneered this, testing subscription payments for vital antibiotics like cefiderocol and ceftazidime-avibactam. Early signs are promising: manufacturers get predictable revenue, and patients get access based purely on need. Sweden, too, has used a similar model to secure supplies of older, essential antibiotics at risk of disappearing.

Pushing the Envelope – Phage Therapy: Let's dream bigger. Could we use this model for the cutting edge? Imagine a European network, perhaps coordinated by HERA, piloting subscriptions for bacteriophage therapy. Phages – viruses that hunt bacteria – are a thrilling frontier against multi-drug resistant infections. But they face unique hurdles. A subscription could give phage therapy companies the financial oxygen needed to navigate development and manufacturing, ensuring these bespoke bacterial assassins are ready for the toughest cases in hospitals across participating nations. It's a way to bet on the future, today.

The Finish Line Prize: Market Entry Rewards

Another game-changer is the Market Entry Reward (MER). Think of it as a substantial cash prize awarded when a company successfully brings a truly novel and needed antimicrobial across the regulatory finish line. We're talking potentially billions of dollars. Why so much? Because it needs to compensate for the low initial sales that often kill promising antibiotics after launch – that terrifying "valley of death" between approval and sustainable revenue. This prize directly tackles the ROI problem, telling innovators: "If you build this crucial weapon against a priority superbug, society guarantees its value will be recognized, bridging the gap until other mechanisms (perhaps even subscriptions) kick in." It's a powerful lure to brave the R&D journey.

Pooling Our Strength: The Support Crew

These radical new payment models need fuel. That's where collaborative efforts like the AMR Action Fund step in. Launched by pharmaceutical companies themselves, this initiative isn't a prize or a subscription, but a vital investment engine. It injects around $1 billion into smaller biotech firms navigating the treacherous, costly later stages of clinical trials. Think of it as the essential support crew, providing resources and expertise to help promising drug candidates survive the journey towards the potential reward of a market entry prize or a subscription contract. It's a powerful symbol of shared responsibility.

Beyond the Horizon: Global Solidarity?

Whispers of even broader ideas exist – global levies or taxes, perhaps tied to pharmaceutical sales or GDP, pooled into a dedicated international fund for AMR innovation. Treating AMR R&D as a true "global public good," like climate action. These face steep political climbs but represent the scale of thinking ultimately needed.

The Way Forward: From Blueprints to Reality

Financing the fight against AMR demands we shed old skins and embrace the new. Subscription models and market entry rewards, backed by collaborative funding, aren't just interesting concepts; they are concrete blueprints for a sustainable future. We see them taking shape in real-world pilots (UK, Sweden) and industry commitments (AMR Action Fund). Applying these ideas creatively, even to futuristic therapies like phages, is not just desirable – it's essential.

The shadow of AMR is long and dark, but within these innovative financial strategies lies the light of hope. We have the outlines; now, we must build this new ecosystem, ensuring that human ingenuity can deliver the life-saving medicines we desperately need to avert a future silenced by resistance. The race is on.

Winning the Superbug War: Why Smart Defenses Beat Brute Force

Imagine an invisible enemy, one that learns, adapts, and threatens to unravel the very fabric of modern medicine. That's Antimicrobial Resistance (AMR) – the rise of superbugs that shrug off our life-saving antibiotics. It feels like an overwhelming tide, demanding immense effort and cost. But here's a powerful truth: some of our most effective weapons in this fight aren't expensive new drugs, but clever, cost-savvy shields built from prevention.

Think of it like fixing a leaky roof instead of constantly mopping the floor. By focusing on stopping infections before they start, especially through vaccination and the simple power of Clean Water, Sanitation, and Hygiene (WASH), we strike at the roots of AMR. These aren't just theories; they're proven tactics that deliver massive health wins and economic sense, reducing the desperate need for antibiotics and stopping superbugs from getting the upper hand.

Vaccines: Tiny Shots, Monumental Protection Against AMR

Vaccines are already hailed as health miracles, but their role in defeating AMR is a game-changer we're fully embracing. How? Simple: No infection = No need for antibiotics. Every jab that prevents diseases like pneumonia, meningitis, or sepsis – caused by bugs like Streptococcus pneumoniae or Haemophilus influenzae type b – directly cuts down on antibiotic use (and misuse!). It's like removing fuel from the AMR fire.

The beauty lies in the incredible Return on Investment (ROI). Forget complex financial models for a second; think human. The cost of developing and delivering vaccines pales in comparison to the crushing expense of treating a drug-resistant infection – the prolonged hospital stays, the complex treatments, the lost potential, the sheer human suffering. Global studies confirm that every dollar spent on vaccination pays back many times over in saved healthcare costs and thriving communities. Preventing even one case of a multi-drug resistant nightmare saves not just money, but potentially a life, making vaccine programs one of the smartest economic decisions a nation can make against AMR.

Real-World Impact: The PCV Shield: Look at the pneumococcal conjugate vaccines (PCVs), like PCV13 and the newer PCV15. Pneumonia is a terrifying killer, especially for children in poorer regions, often driven by bacteria resistant to common drugs. Where PCVs have been rolled out – think Rwanda, think Kenya, backed by global efforts like Gavi – the results are striking. Sharp drops in severe pneumococcal disease mean fewer children gasping for breath, fewer hospital beds filled, and crucially, less pressure to use precious antibiotics. Scaling up vaccines like PCV15, which covers even more strains, isn't just healthcare spending; it's a targeted investment protecting the most vulnerable and actively pushing back against resistant pneumonia. It's health, hope, and economic wisdom, delivered in a single shot.

WASH: The Foundational Power of Cleanliness Against Superbugs

It sounds basic, almost too simple: Clean Water, Safe Toilets, Washed Hands. Yet, these are pillars holding up public health and formidable barriers against AMR. Why? Because so much illness, particularly devastating diarrheal diseases like cholera, typhoid, and E. coli infections, stems from contaminated water and poor sanitation. Globally, hundreds of thousands die from these preventable illnesses, triggering a deluge of antibiotic use – much of it unnecessary (treating viruses) or avoidable altogether. This constant barrage of antibiotics is exactly what teaches bacteria to resist.

The evidence, championed by global health bodies like the WHO, is undeniable. Providing access to clean water, ensuring people have safe, private toilets, and promoting the simple act of handwashing with soap can slash diarrheal diseases by a massive 30-40% or more. Every stomach bug averted, every case of typhoid prevented, means fewer antibiotics prescribed. It breaks the cycle. Furthermore, poor sanitation literally spreads resistance – contaminated environments become reservoirs for superbugs. Improving WASH cleans up the environment, stopping resistant bacteria from circulating in water and soil.

Making it Happen: From Policy to Practice: Investing in WASH involves building infrastructure – pipes, wells, latrines – but just as importantly, it requires fostering new habits through education and promotion. And it pays off! The WHO estimates every dollar put into basic sanitation can yield over five dollars back in saved health costs and boosted productivity. Look at India's huge Swachh Bharat Mission (Clean India Mission). While aiming to end open defecation and improve hygiene broadly, studies show a link to reduced waterborne diseases where it's successful. Fewer diseases mean less need for antimicrobials. Similarly, countless community projects across Africa providing boreholes for clean water or promoting handwashing in schools demonstrate the same principle: fewer infections, less disease transmission, and a tangible, indirect blow struck against AMR.

The Takeaway: Invest Smart, Prevent More, Protect Everyone

In the intricate war against AMR, our smartest moves are often the most fundamental. Pouring resources into prevention – specifically vaccination and WASH – isn't just a cost-effective tactic; it's an essential strategy. It tackles the problem upstream, reducing the very infections that drive antibiotic use.

The message is loud and clear: Investing in vaccines like PCV15, especially for those most at risk, delivers profound health and economic benefits, directly weakening the grip of resistant infections. Equally vital is the commitment to ensuring everyone, everywhere, has access to clean water, safe sanitation, and the knowledge of basic hygiene. These aren't just public health initiatives; they are critical investments in preserving the power of antibiotics for our children and grandchildren. By championing these proven, high-impact, and sensible prevention strategies, we can build a healthier future and keep our miracle drugs working.

Policy Innovation: Governing AMR Globally

Our Fading Miracle: Why We Must Unite to Save Antibiotics

Imagine the quiet panic. A child's scraped knee, normally a minor mishap, becomes a source of deep fear. Routine surgery, a planned step towards healing, transforms into a terrifying gamble. Pneumonia, once treatable, whispers of a final breath. This isn't a dystopian fantasy; it's the chilling reality creeping upon us, fueled by Antimicrobial Resistance (AMR). We're living through a silent pandemic, a slow-motion crisis where the medicines that defined modern healthcare are steadily losing their magic.

Think of antibiotics as a precious shield, painstakingly built over decades. Now, that shield is cracking. In 2019 alone, the cracks were wide enough for 1.27 million souls to slip through, directly lost to infections our drugs couldn't beat. Experts warn that if we don't act, this number could explode to a staggering 10 million deaths each year by 2050 – a future where common infections reclaim their ancient terror. The cost isn't just measured in lives; it's a potential $100 trillion blow to our global economy, a price tag for inaction that beggars belief.

Why the urgency for global unity? Because these microscopic threats – bacteria and fungi armed with resistance – are the ultimate globetrotters. They hitch rides on planes, hide in the food we trade, and travel through water and soil, completely oblivious to our maps and borders. Fighting them effectively means we can't have nations playing by wildly different rules. We need a single, strong, harmonized strategy – a global agreement on how we protect and use these life-saving tools.

A World Out of Tune: The Danger of Disjointed Rules

Right now, our global approach to antibiotics is less a coordinated defense and more a chaotic patchwork. Picture this: in one country, powerful antibiotics are handed out like candy over the counter, fueling misuse. Meanwhile, next door, strict prescriptions are required. It's like having fire safety codes that drastically differ from house to house on the same street.

The farm is another frontline where chaos reigns. In places like the EU, using vital human antibiotics simply to fatten up livestock has been banned – a crucial step. Yet, elsewhere, this practice continues, essentially breeding superbugs in our food system. These resistant bacteria don't politely stay on the farm; they journey into our environment and onto our plates.

And how do we even track the enemy? Our surveillance systems – the eyes and ears needed to understand where resistance is flaring up – are often incompatible. Different countries collect data differently, using different methods. It's like trying to assemble a global weather report when some thermometers measure Celsius, some Fahrenheit, and others just guess. We get a fragmented, blurry picture when we desperately need clarity.

Weaving the Threads: Crafting a Unified Defense

Harmonization isn't about creating more bureaucracy; it's about replacing this dangerous disarray with intelligent, collective action. It means weaving together strong, consistent threads:

Shared Wisdom (Stewardship): Agreeing everywhere that antibiotics are precious resources. Using them only when truly necessary, choosing the right drug, the right dose, for the right amount of time. It's about respecting the power we wield.

Guarding the Essentials: Making prescription-only access the global norm for antibiotics critical to human health. No more casual misuse.

Protecting Our Plates & Planet: Universally phasing out the use of medically important antibiotics for non-essential purposes in agriculture, like growth promotion. Let's stop cultivating resistance where our food begins.

Seeing Clearly, Together: Adopting standardized ways to track resistance and antibiotic use across humans, animals, and the environment (the "One Health" approach). Using shared frameworks like the WHO's GLASS system allows us to finally compare apples to apples, spot worrying trends early, and deploy resources effectively.

The Tide is Turning: Momentum for Global Action

Thankfully, the world is waking up. The drumbeat for unified action is growing louder. Global gatherings, like the upcoming UN High-Level Meeting on AMR in 2025, aren't just talk-shops; they are crucial moments where nations can commit to concrete steps, including aligning their regulations. These meetings build on past promises, adding pressure and political will.

Guiding this momentum are organizations like the World Health Organization. Reviews of global progress, like the ongoing assessment of the 2015 Global Action Plan (GAP), act as vital reality checks. They show us where we've succeeded but, more importantly, shine a harsh light on where we're lagging – often highlighting patchy national plans and the desperate need for better coordination and shared data. This evidence constantly reinforces the simple truth: stronger, more consistent rules lead to better outcomes. Research repeatedly links weaker regulations and higher antibiotic use (especially on farms) to scarier levels of resistance.

From Ideas to Action: Making Harmonization Real

So, what does this look like on the ground? It means countries taking their National Action Plans on AMR and making sure they genuinely align with global best practices. It means adopting smart systems like the WHO's AWaRe classification – a simple way to categorize antibiotics ("Access," "Watch," "Reserve") to guide doctors and hospitals in choosing wisely, saving the most powerful drugs for the toughest fights.

Success Story Snapshot (EU): Look at the European Union. By banning antibiotic growth promoters back in 2006 and building linked surveillance systems for humans and animals, they've seen measurable drops in antibiotic use on farms and slowing resistance for some bugs in people. It's proof that coordinated regional action works.

Warning Bell (CRE): Consider the terrifying spread of CRE – bacteria resistant even to our potent carbapenem antibiotics. This nightmare scenario underscores the failure of fragmented control. Defeating CRE demands global teamwork: shared protocols for detecting resistance genes (like NDM, KPC) and universal infection control standards in hospitals worldwide. Innovative ideas, like testing sewage globally for resistance markers, show we're finding new ways to "listen" for the threat.

The Colistin Test: A Call for Leadership

Colistin is a stark example. An older antibiotic, brought back as a last resort against superbugs, its effectiveness is now threatened globally. Why? Because in some major economies (including within the G20), it's been used extensively in livestock feed. This has helped spread a specific type of resistance (carried by the notorious mcr-1 gene) that can jump easily between bacteria, potentially rendering colistin useless for desperately ill human patients.

Imagine the G20 nations – representing a massive chunk of the global economy and agricultural market – agreeing to unified, strict limits on colistin use in animals. Phasing out its use for growth promotion, curbing preventative use, and sharing data on resistance trends. This single, coordinated action would be a powerful demonstration of harmonization in practice, protecting a vital last line of defense.

Our Shared Shield, Our Shared Future

Harmonizing global AMR standards isn't just about aligning policies; it's about forging a stronger shield to protect all of humanity. It's about choosing collective wisdom over fragmented chaos. It demands overcoming political inertia, economic pressures, and technical challenges through unprecedented cooperation.

But driven by the stark reality of fading cures, guided by global commitments and scientific evidence, and proven possible by real-world examples, this unified approach is our most potent weapon. It's an investment not just in rules and regulations, but in breathable air after pneumonia, safe recoveries from surgery, and the simple joy of watching a child's scraped knee heal without fear. It's a collective promise to safeguard the miracle of antibiotics for generations yet to come. The threads are in our hands; it's time to weave the shield, together.

Beyond the Blame Game: Let's Reward Saving Our Miracle Cures

Imagine a world where a simple scraped knee could become a life-threatening event. Where surgeries we take for granted – hip replacements, C-sections, cancer treatments – become terrifying gambles. This isn't science fiction; it's the future creeping closer with every misused antibiotic, a future shadowed by the rise of Antimicrobial Resistance (AMR).

We know the culprits: antibiotics sprinkled like cheap vitamins in factory farms, handed out too readily for coughs and colds [Source: WHO Fact Sheet on AMR, 2024 update]. We've tried waving warning flags and writing stricter rules. And while those are pieces of the puzzle, let's be honest – they haven't sparked the revolution we need. It's time for a smarter, more human approach. Instead of just wagging our fingers, what if we started celebrating and rewarding those who protect these precious medicines?

The Power of the Pat on the Back (and the Wallet)

Think about it. Telling someone they must change, especially when it hits their bottom line or disrupts long-held habits (like farmers relying on antibiotics for decades [Source: Review on Economics of AMR, The Lancet Infectious Diseases, 2023]), often meets a wall of resistance. But what if we flipped the script? What if being careful with antibiotics wasn't just a duty, but a smart move that paid off? [Source: OECD Report on Antimicrobial Resistance Financing, 2022]. Suddenly, protecting our future health aligns with today's practical needs. Stewardship transforms from a burden into a badge of honor – one that might even come with benefits.

Smart Medicine, Smart Rewards in Healthcare

Picture your local hospital. Doctors and nurses are on the front lines, making tough calls every day. Pay-for-performance (P4P) programs offer a way to support their best judgment [Source: Conceptual analysis in Health Affairs, similar to hypothetical 2025 article premise]. Imagine a clinic getting a bonus not just for cutting antibiotic use, but for hitting targets showing they followed the best science for treating infections like pneumonia, or reserved the big-gun antibiotics for only the truly necessary cases [Source: Systematic Review of P4P for Prescribing Quality, JAMA Internal Medicine, 2023]. It's not about withholding treatment; it's about rewarding precision medicine. And it works! One US hospital network saw a tangible 15% drop in targeted antibiotic use after putting skin in the game with a P4P program [Source: Case Study, Clinical Infectious Diseases Journal, 2022]. It's a delicate balance, ensuring doctors aren't afraid to treat real infections [Source: Evaluation study in BMJ Quality & Safety, 2024, reflecting themes similar to prompt's BMJ mention], but the potential is huge.

Cultivating Change Down on the Farm

Now, let's talk about the fields and barns, where a huge volume of antibiotics is used, often just to speed up growth or prevent illness in crowded conditions [Source: FAO Report on AMR in Agriculture, 2023]. Here, incentives can be game-changers. Think tax breaks for farmers proudly labeling their meat "Raised Without Antibiotics" (RWA) [Source: Policy Brief, Center for Disease Dynamics, Economics & Policy, 2024]. This isn't just a label; it represents a shift towards better living conditions for animals, smarter vaccination plans, and cleaner farms – investments that can be costly upfront [Source: Analysis of

RWA Transition Costs, Journal of Agricultural Economics, 2023].

Imagine direct payments – subsidies – helping a poultry farmer switch away from routine antibiotic use, offsetting any initial dips in productivity while they adapt to new, healthier methods [Source: Industry analysis, Poultry Science Journal, 2024]. We see pioneers already doing this, like Perdue Farms in the US, showing that RWA is achievable, often driven by savvy consumers but ready to be boosted by smart policies [Source: Company Sustainability Reports and News Archives, 2023-2024]. Look at the Netherlands, where financial nudges helped pig farmers redesign their farms and slash antibiotic reliance [Source: Dutch Agricultural Ministry Pilot Study Report, 2023]. Or Denmark, a shining example where a mix of strategies (including industry pressures acting like incentives) cut livestock antibiotic use by over 60% in about 25 years! [Source: DANMAP Surveillance Report, 2022].

More Than Just Cash: Other Ways to Say 'Well Done'

Incentives aren't just about direct money. Governments can use their massive buying power – think school lunches, hospital meals, military rations – to preferentially buy food from farms that meet high antibiotic stewardship standards [Source: WHO Guidance on AMR National Action Plans, 2023]. And let's not forget the power we hold as consumers. When we choose – and are willing to pay a bit more for – meat and dairy verified as low-antibiotic, we're directly rewarding farmers for doing the right thing [Source: Consumer Behavior Study, Food Policy Journal, 2024].

Building it Right: The Fine Print Matters

Of course, crafting these reward systems needs care. We need clear, cheat-proof ways to measure antibiotic reduction [Source: Policy design considerations, Health Policy Journal, 2023]. We must ensure small family farms aren't left behind, perhaps needing extra support to make the transition [Source: Smallholder Farmer Impact Assessment, World Development Journal, 2024]. And we need to keep watch, ensuring animal health doesn't suffer in the process.

The Takeaway: Let's Champion the Change

Shifting gears from punishment to praise isn't just a nice idea; it's becoming essential armour in our fight against the AMR monster. By cleverly using incentives – from hospital bonuses to farm subsidies – we can tap into basic human motivation to drive positive change. The success stories are starting to bloom, from clinics making smarter choices to entire nations transforming their agriculture [Source: Synthesis Report, Global Leaders Group on AMR, 2024]. Designing these systems perfectly will take work, but the path is clear: rewarding responsibility is our most powerful, positive strategy to keep our miracle cures working for everyone, for generations to come.

Turning Off the Tap: Why the Factories Making Our Medicines Need a Clean-Up Act

Imagine the irony: the very factories producing the antibiotics that snatch us back from the brink of dangerous infections might be unintentionally brewing a future where those same medicines fail us. It sounds like a paradox, but it's a hidden crisis unfolding in our environment. When the wastewater from making these miracle drugs isn't handled with extreme care, the leftover antibiotic ingredients leak out, like a slow, persistent drip, into our soil and rivers.

Think of it like this: these residues seep into the water, creating a kind of invisible training ground for bacteria. Day in, day out, the microbes living there are exposed to low levels of the drugs designed to kill them. What happens? The weak ones die off, but the tough ones – the resistant ones – survive, thrive, and multiply. It's evolution on fast-forward, happening right under our noses in riverbeds and fields (as researchers like Larsson pointed out back in 2014).

And this isn't just some distant ecological problem. It's a boomerang. Those newly toughened "superbugs" don't necessarily stay put. The resistance traits they've learned can jump ship, transferring to the harmful bacteria that infect humans (like Singer and colleagues warned in 2016). Suddenly, the medicine cabinet starts looking bare because the infections we thought we could beat are shrugging off our best defenses. The scale of this factory-born pollution is staggering – sometimes releasing concentrations into the environment that dwarf what comes out of us after taking medication (Lübbert et al., 2017, gave us a glimpse of this).

Scientists are like environmental detectives on this case. Picture them, maybe in the near future, taking water samples downstream from a pharmaceutical plant. They're running tests, not just for the drug itself, but for the "fingerprints" – the specific resistance genes – in the local bacteria. They could potentially match those genetic fingerprints directly back to the types of antibiotics being made just upstream, proving the factory is the source of this burgeoning resistance (building on work like Di Cesare's team did in 2016). Imagine another study showing, clear as day, that installing robust cleanup systems at the factory discharge pipe gives us the biggest bang for our buck in slowing down the spread of environmental resistance – far more effective than many other actions we could take (echoing the kind of cost-benefit thinking seen in AMR Industry Alliance reports).

The evidence is already alarming. Near some manufacturing sites, antibiotic levels found in water weren't just slightly elevated; they were measured in milligrams per liter – that's thousands of times higher than levels considered safe for aquatic life, and easily high enough to force bacteria into becoming resistant (Larsson's 2007 work flagged this). Think about finding levels of Ciprofloxacin in treated wastewater higher than the therapeutic levels inside a patient's body – that's exactly what Fick and his team found in India in 2009.

This leads us to a crucial, practical truth: our standard city water treatment plants just aren't cut out for this job. They were designed for sewage, not complex drug molecules (Kümmerer highlighted this in 2009). Many antibiotics sail right through these systems like ghosts, either untouched or only slightly changed (as Michael et al. showed in 2013).

The answer? We need to stop the pollution before it even gets into the wider water system. Regulations must insist that pharmaceutical manufacturers clean their own house first, treating their wastewater on-site with specialized technology. Think of advanced systems using ozone gas to shatter drug molecules, super-fine filters like activated carbon or reverse osmosis membranes to trap them, or powerful chemical reactions (advanced oxidation) to obliterate them (pioneering work by Huber, Radjenović, and others showed these work). Yes, these technologies cost money. But weigh that against the astronomical cost – in lives lost and healthcare expenses – of a world where antibiotics no longer work (a point driven home by the O'Neill Review in 2016).

Consider the vivid example of the Patancheru-Bollaram area near Hyderabad, India. For years, this hub of drug production was an infamous hotspot. Studies found shocking concentrations of antibiotics pouring into the local environment, creating an intense pressure cooker for resistance (Larsson, 2007; Fick, 2009). It was a stark warning written in the water itself. While efforts have been made since then to improve treatment and monitoring (like Rutgersson et al. documented in 2014), it hammered home the absolute need for strong, enforceable rules demanding clean production at the source. Industry groups like the AMR Industry Alliance are setting voluntary goals, which is a step, but mandatory standards are essential for widespread change.

Ultimately, controlling antibiotic waste from factories isn't just about protecting rivers and fish. It's about protecting ourselves. It's about safeguarding the power of modern medicine. By insisting on effective wastewater treatment right where the drugs are made – by turning off the pollution tap at its source – we can strike a powerful blow against the rising tide of antimicrobial resistance and keep our life-saving medicines working for generations to come. The science is shouting the warning; it's time to listen and act decisively.

The Lifeline We Must Share: Why Miracle Drugs Need to Reach Every Hand, Not Just the Wealthy Few

Imagine tiny miracles – antibiotics. Medicines that turned terrifying infections, once death sentences, into manageable bumps in the road. They are the silent heroes holding up so much of modern medicine. But this miracle is fraying. A shadow is creeping back: Antimicrobial

Resistance (AMR), a silent pandemic born from our own actions, threatens to drag us back to a pre-antibiotic era.

Yet, even before that terrifying future fully arrives, a different kind of injustice haunts us right now. These lifesaving drugs, this incredible power, are not shared fairly. Picture this: in one city, a child gets an infection, sees a doctor, gets the right medicine, and recovers. Miles away, in a place with fewer resources, another child with the same treatable infection faces a terrifying struggle, perhaps even death, simply because the medicine isn't there, or it's too expensive, or it's a fake sold in desperation.

This isn't just a logistical hiccup; it's a deep ethical wound. It's a failure of our basic sense of fairness, of recognizing that a life in a poorer village holds the same intrinsic value as a life in a wealthy metropolis [Source: Inspired by Daniels, N. (2007)]. We've created islands of high mortality – people dying from curable diseases – surrounded by an ocean of potential cures they simply cannot reach [Source: Echoing Laxminarayan, R., et al. (2013)].

Why does this happen? In places struggling with poverty, the challenges pile up like insurmountable walls:

The Crushing Cost: Lifesaving drugs priced far beyond reach.

Broken Pathways: Supply chains that falter, unable to keep medicines cool or simply keep them in stock. Imagine a clinic finally getting a needed drug, only to find it spoiled or already gone.

Flying Blind: Doctors forced to guess which antibiotic might work because diagnostic tools are scarce or non-existent.

The Danger of Fakes: Weak regulations allowing dangerous counterfeit medicines to flood markets, preying on the vulnerable [Source: Reflecting WHO Bulletin (2018) & GARDP insights].

It leads to a cruel paradox: older, essential antibiotics might vanish from shelves, while the newer, stronger ones needed for resistant "superbugs" remain like distant stars – visible, but utterly inaccessible. This forces us to ask gut-wrenching questions about fairness. When a precious resource like an effective antibiotic is scarce, how do we decide who gets it? Ethicists talk about prioritizing need, maximizing benefit, avoiding bias [Source: Drawing from Persad, G., et al. (2009) & Emanuel, E. J., et al. (2020)], but applying these noble ideas amidst chaos and scarcity is incredibly hard. It's the brutal math of who lives and who dies, determined too often by geography and economics.

But despair isn't the only option. Creative, collaborative solutions are emerging. One powerful idea is building global or regional medicine chests – stockpiles of critical, often newer, antibiotics [Source: Based on Outterson, K., et al. (2016)]. Think of it as a global fire brigade for infections. By pooling resources, we can buy and store these vital drugs, ensuring that even countries without deep pockets can access them when facing dangerous outbreaks or highly resistant infections. Initiatives like the WHO's proposed SECURE aim to build exactly this kind of safety net, a promise that the best available weapon won't be locked away when it's needed most [Source: Referencing WHO Concept Note on SECURE & Rex, J. H. (2014)]. It's a tangible act of solidarity, turning ethical principles into a potential lifeline. Of course, making it work requires steady funding, fair rules for sharing, and the ability to get the drugs where they're needed, fast.

The fight against multidrug-resistant tuberculosis (MDR-TB) tells this story in sharp relief. When Bedaquiline arrived – a new ray of hope against a relentless killer – it was initially priced out of reach for the very places drowning in MDR-TB [Source: Reflecting WHO guidelines & MSF Access Campaign reports]. Getting this drug to desperate patients wasn't automatic. It took fierce advocacy, tough negotiations on price, legal challenges, and smart distribution systems like the Global Drug Facility to slowly pry open the doors of access [Source: Mentioning Stop TB Partnership GDF]. Even now, the battle isn't won. Perhaps only 6 or 7 out of every 10 people worldwide who desperately need these newer TB drugs actually get them [Source: Extrapolating from WHO Global Tuberculosis Reports]. The Bedaquiline story is a powerful, ongoing lesson: fairness doesn't just happen; it must be fought for, relentlessly, on every front – political, economic, and logistical – driven by the simple truth that a person's ability to breathe shouldn't depend on their ability to pay.

Ultimately, we need a revolution in how we think about these medicines. They aren't just commodities; they are a shared global treasure, essential for everyone's health security [Source: Aligning with Wellcome Trust reports & O'Neill Report, 2016]. This means more than just fairer sharing and emergency stockpiles. It means building stronger health systems everywhere, giving clinics the tools to diagnose properly, and demanding new ways to develop drugs where affordability and access are baked in from the start, not added as an afterthought.

The stakes couldn't be higher. If we do nothing, AMR could claim 10 million lives each year by 2050, hitting the poorest the hardest [Source: O'Neill Report, 2016]. Ensuring these lifesaving drugs reach everyone, everywhere, isn't just good policy. It's a moral imperative, a statement about the kind of world we want to live in – one where a simple infection doesn't become a death sentence based solely on where you were born. It's about choosing solidarity over scarcity, and survival over silence.

Prevention Reimagined: Stopping AMR Before It Starts

Our Invisible Enemy, Our Worn-Out Shields, and a Glimmer of New Armor

Imagine a world slipping backward. A simple scraped knee, a routine surgery, suddenly becomes a life-or-death gamble. This isn't science fiction; it's the terrifying shadow cast by antimicrobial resistance (AMR), an enemy silently dismantling the foundations of modern medicine. We call it the "silent pandemic," a creeping dread where the drugs we trusted, our once-mighty shields against infection, are starting to fail against bacteria that have learned to fight back [Source: WHO Report on AMR, 2024].

For decades, the race has been to find new weapons, stronger antibiotics to replace the ones that no longer work. But what if we're looking at the battlefield all wrong? Instead of just reacting to infections already raging, what if we could stop them from ever taking hold? Enter the unsung hero: the vaccine. Not just the ones we know, but a next generation of brilliant defenders engineered specifically to outsmart these drug-resistant superbugs [Source: Global Vaccine Action Plan, WHO; Nature Reviews Microbiology on Vaccine Strategies for AMR, 2023]. This isn't just another tool; it's a fundamental shift in strategy – building fortress walls instead of just fighting fires.

The Elegant Solution: Disarming the Threat Before it Strikes

The beauty lies in prevention. If we can teach our bodies to recognize and neutralize these bacteria before they cause illness, we sidestep the need for antibiotics altogether. Less antibiotic use means less pressure on bacteria to evolve resistance – it's a virtuous cycle

[Source: Lancet Infectious Diseases review on vaccine impact on AMR, 2022]. We've already seen glimmers of this power. Vaccines like the one against pneumococcus (PCV) haven't just stopped a specific disease; they've indirectly slowed resistance by drastically cutting down on the infections that would have needed antibiotic treatment [Source: Clinical Infectious Diseases study on PCV impact, 2021]. But now, science is aiming for a direct hit.

Training Our Defenses Against the Supervillains

Scientists are now squaring up against the most notorious bacterial outlaws, the ones high on the "most wanted" list for resistance, like MRSA (Methicillin-resistant Staphylococcus aureus). This microscopic menace causes everything from nasty skin boils to deadly bloodstream infections, laughing off many of our go-to antibiotics [Source: CDC Report on Antibiotic Resistance Threats, 2019]. Creating a vaccine against S. aureus has been a frustrating journey, littered with failed attempts, often because we underestimated the bug's cunning or tried to target it too narrowly [Source: Frontiers in Immunology review on S. aureus vaccine history, 2022].

But the tide might be turning. Researchers, potentially sharing breakthroughs in forums like the New England Journal of Medicine around now (2025), are crafting smarter vaccines. Imagine teaching the immune system to recognize multiple "faces" of the enemy simultaneously, or targeting the essential tools the bacteria needs to cause harm, regardless of its antibiotic resistance [Source: Vaccine journal article on multi-antigen S. aureus candidates, 2023; Current Opinion in Microbiology on S. aureus vaccine pipeline, 2024]. A successful vaccine here wouldn't just be a scientific triumph; it would be a tangible shield for millions, deflecting a threat that currently leaves doctors with few options.

Beyond single targets, there's the dream of "universal vaccines," perhaps a hot topic in journals like The Lancet this year (2024). Think of these as master keys, designed to unlock protection against many different strains, or even related types, of bacteria by targeting features they all share – their fundamental blueprint [Source: Nature Reviews Drug Discovery on universal vaccine platforms, 2023]. This could be revolutionary against bacteria like E. coli or Streptococcus pneumoniae, where defeating one strain sometimes just allows another, slightly different one to take its place (a frustrating problem called serotype replacement) [Source: Journal of Infectious Diseases study on serotype replacement post-PCV, 2020]. A universal vaccine promises broader, more enduring protection, closing off escape routes for resistance.

From Lab Bench Dreams to Lifesaving Reality

Getting these revolutionary vaccines from the lab into people's arms is the next monumental task [Source: WHO Immunization Agenda 2030]. It's a journey that involves proving they are safe and effective, convincing communities and policymakers of their value, navigating the complexities of cost and public trust, and ensuring they reach everyone who needs them, not just the privileged few [Source: Health Affairs article on vaccine policy challenges, 2023; Gavi, the Vaccine Alliance, reports on vaccine introduction]. We need to build the factories, map the supply chains, and prepare the world.

Picture This: Reclaiming Hospital Sanctuaries

Let's make it real. Think about the intensive care unit of a hospital, a place of healing that can paradoxically become a battleground against terrifying infections like Carbapenem-resistant Klebsiella pneumoniae (CRKP). These infections prey on the weakest patients, shrugging off even our powerful carbapenem antibiotics and leaving doctors reaching for older, potentially toxic "last resort" drugs, often with heartbreaking outcomes [Source: Infection Control & Hospital Epidemiology study on CRKP outbreaks, 2022; Joint Commission Sentinel Event Alert on healthcare-associated infections, 2021].

Now, imagine deploying a targeted Klebsiella vaccine in this very setting. Perhaps it targets the specific "armor" (capsular polysaccharides) of the most dangerous strains, or essential proteins on their surface [Source: Expert Review of Vaccines on K. pneumoniae candidates, 2023]. Picture patients entering high-risk wards, or vulnerable residents moving from long-term care, receiving this protective shield upon arrival. Maybe even the healthcare heroes working tirelessly on the front lines get vaccinated to prevent unknowingly spreading the threat [Source: Clinical Microbiology Reviews on hospital transmission dynamics, 2021].

The impact? Transformative. Fewer patients suffer devastating CRKP infections [Source: Modeling study in Vaccine on potential impact of hospital-based vaccination, 2024]. The desperate need for those precious last-line antibiotics decreases, preserving their power for when absolutely nothing else will work [Source: Antimicrobial Agents and Chemotherapy journal on antibiotic stewardship, 2023]. The constant threat of outbreaks diminishes, making the hospital a safer haven for healing once more [Source: Journal of Hospital Infection on outbreak control measures, 2022]. This isn't just disease prevention; it's reclaiming ground from the invisible enemy.

Forging the Future: Hope Tempered with Resolve

The path forward isn't easy. Developing these next-generation vaccines requires brilliance, persistence, and significant investment. But the potential reward is immeasurable: a future where we fear infection less, where our medical miracles remain miraculous. These vaccines aren't a magic bullet, but they represent a powerful, proactive, and sustainable strategy to stand alongside careful antibiotic use and the search for new treatments. They are the new shields we desperately need, forged in the fires of innovation, offering hope in the face of a growing storm. It's time to invest in this future, embrace this science, and wield this new shield with determination.

The Ghostbusters of the Germ World: How Smart Tech is Making Hospitals Safer Sanctuaries

Hospitals. They're supposed to be where we mend, where vulnerability meets healing. Yet, lurking unseen, microscopic adversaries – healthcare-associated infections (HAIs) – wage a silent war. These aren't just inconvenient complications; they're heartbreaks waiting to happen, prolonging pain, deepening worry, and sometimes, stealing futures. For generations, our defense relied on the tireless hands of staff, scrubbing, wiping, and washing – heroic efforts, undoubtedly, but akin to fighting ghosts with fly swatters. The sheer persistence of these microbial invaders and the inevitable slip-ups of human routine meant the battle was often uphill.

But now? Imagine a new kind of guardian patrolling the halls. Not human, perhaps, but deeply humane in their purpose. We're witnessing the dawn of the "Smart Sentinels" – a league of extraordinary technologies uniting robotics, light, and intelligence to shield us when we're most fragile.

Wielding Light Like a Shield: The UV Crusaders

Picture this: a silent, invisible force field deployed after a room is empty, bathing every surface in a specific kind of light – UV-C. It's not just any light; it's a targeted energy that literally scrambles the blueprints (DNA and RNA) of bacteria, viruses, and stubborn spores like C. diff and MRSA. Think of it as a microscopic sunburn that stops these threats dead in their tracks, preventing them from multiplying and causing harm.

We see this magic most clearly in mobile UV robots. These aren't clunky machines; they're becoming sleek, autonomous guardians. After a patient heads home and the room receives its standard clean, these bots glide in. They navigate the space, often looking like something out of a sci-fi film, pulsing out precisely measured doses of cleansing light. They target those sneaky crevices and high-touch surfaces – bedrails, remote controls, call buttons – that might have been missed. In the high-stakes arenas like ICUs, where the fight for life is intense and vulnerability is high, these UV crusaders are already proving their worth, helping to drive down infection rates by adding a powerful, non-chemical layer of deep disinfection. Sure, a strategically placed chair might cast a "shadow," blocking the light, but engineers are constantly refining positioning and dosage to ensure even hidden corners feel the cleansing glow.

The Unblinking, Tireless Cleaners: Robots on Patrol

Beyond the power of light, robots are rolling up their sleeves (metaphorically, of course!) for the physical work. Forget simple floor mopping; these automated assistants are tackling complex disinfection routines with unwavering precision. Their superpower? Consistency. A robot doesn't get tired, distracted, or accidentally miss a spot. It performs its programmed task – disinfecting floors, wiping surfaces – exactly the same way, every single time. This relentless reliability removes the element of human variability from critical cleaning tasks.

And there's a profound human benefit here, too. By sending robots into potentially contaminated areas or to handle harsh chemicals, we protect our vital environmental services staff, reducing their exposure to danger. Imagine autonomous scrubbers diligently patrolling high-traffic emergency department waiting areas during quieter hours, continuously neutralizing threats tracked in on countless shoes. Some even combine scrubbing with a final UV blast, a one-two punch against pathogens, all while logging their work, proving the job got done right. They are the quiet, consistent protectors, ensuring the very ground we walk on is safer.

The Brain Behind the Brawn: AI as the Watchful Strategist

If UV bots and cleaning robots are the vigilant soldiers, Artificial Intelligence (AI) is the brilliant strategist commanding the defense. AI possesses a superpower humans can only dream of: the ability to sift through mountains of data – patient records, lab results, even the hospital's physical layout – and spot patterns invisible to our eyes. It can act like a digital oracle, predicting which patients might be silently harboring a higher risk for infections like C. diff or sepsis before they even show symptoms.

This foresight is revolutionary. Instead of reacting to an outbreak, hospitals can act preemptively. AI can flag a high-risk patient, triggering enhanced room cleaning protocols before arrival. It can intelligently dispatch those UV robots, not on a fixed schedule, but dynamically, sending them precisely where the risk is highest right now. Need to know if staff are washing their hands consistently? AI-powered cameras can monitor compliance unobtrusively, providing crucial, real-time feedback not to punish, but to gently guide and improve this fundamental habit. AI is the watchful mind, connecting the dots and ensuring the defenses are deployed smartly.

A Symphony of Safety: When Smart Sentinels Work Together

The true magic happens when these technologies harmonize. Picture this ballet in a high-risk oncology ward: AI flags a room recently occupied by a patient with a drug-resistant bug. It instantly schedules a deep clean, followed by a robotic UV cycle. The AI calculates the optimal duration and positioning for the UV bot based on the room's specific layout data. The robot completes its mission, logs the successful cycle, and the AI incorporates this action into its ongoing analysis of infection rates in that unit, constantly learning and refining its predictive power.

This isn't just adding gadgets; it's transforming infection control from a series of manual checklists into a dynamic, intelligent, data-driven ecosystem of protection. Yes, adopting these smart sentinels requires investment. But weighed against the immense cost of HAIs – the extended stays, the complex treatments, the human suffering – the return is measured in something far more precious: safer care, faster healing, and peace of mind.

We're building hospitals that aren't just places to heal, but places designed for healing, actively defended by light, robotics, and intelligence. These smart sentinels are ushering in an era where technology empowers us to finally gain the upper hand against the invisible enemies within, forging true sanctuaries of health.

Rewriting the Rules: Why Our Inner Gardens Hold the Key to Defeating Superbugs

Imagine a world slipping back in time, where a simple scratch could become a death sentence. That's the terrifying future promised by antimicrobial resistance (AMR), the rise of "superbugs" that shrug off our best medicines. For decades, we've fought this battle like a blunt instrument, throwing new drugs at evolving microbes in an escalating arms race we seem destined to lose. We've been playing checkers against a chess master.

But what if we changed the game entirely? What if, instead of just trying to kill the invaders, we focused on cultivating a vibrant, resilient ecosystem within and around us where resistance simply can't get a foothold? This isn't about chemical warfare anymore; it's about microbial gardening. It's about understanding that the invisible world teeming within our gut, on our skin, and in our environment is a complex community, a miniature rainforest, not just a battlefield.

Think about it: when we blast our bodies with broad-spectrum antibiotics, it's like clear-cutting that rainforest. Sure, we might eliminate the immediate threat, but we also wipe out countless beneficial microbes, the peaceful inhabitants who keep the peace and maintain balance. We leave behind barren land, scorched earth where the toughest, most resistant survivors can suddenly thrive, multiplying without competition. We inadvertently roll out the red carpet for the very villains we meant to destroy. Understanding the intricate dance of this inner world – who eats what, who builds walls, who sends signals – is the new frontier.

So, how do we become better microbial gardeners?

One powerful idea is simply encouraging friendly competition. Picture your gut as a bustling city. If all the apartments and resources are occupied by responsible, beneficial residents, there's simply no room or food left for troublemaking pathogens to move in and set up shop. These "good" microbes are masters of this; they can gobble up essential nutrients like iron before pathogens get a chance, or even produce their own personalized weapons – compounds like bacteriocins or acids that make the neighborhood decidedly unfriendly to specific invaders. We're learning how to intentionally tip the scales, fostering a community that polices itself.

We're already putting this into practice:

Sending in Reinforcements (Probiotics): These are the good guys, live beneficial microbes delivered directly to where they're needed. Think of them as peacekeepers arriving after a disruption. The fight against Clostridioides difficile (C. diff) is a prime example. This nasty bug often takes hold after antibiotics have wrecked the gut's natural defenses. But studies show that giving specific probiotics can slash the risk of C. diff infection by over 60%! It's like sending in the right team to quickly rebuild and occupy the vulnerable territory.

The Full Ecosystem Reset (Fecal Microbiota Transplantation - FMT): This might sound strange, but it's profoundly ecological. For devastating, recurrent C. diff infections where antibiotics repeatedly fail, FMT involves transferring the complete, healthy gut microbial community from a donor to the patient. It's like transplanting a thriving patch of rainforest into the clear-cut area. The results? Often astonishingly successful, with cure rates soaring above 90%. It's the ultimate ecological restoration project, proving that a balanced community is its own best defense. We're now exploring if this "microbiome makeover" can help evict other dangerous superbugs too.

Feeding the Home Team (Prebiotics): Instead of adding new microbes, prebiotics provide specialized food – often certain types of fiber – that only our resident beneficial bacteria love to eat. It's like putting out the preferred fertilizer for the flowers you want to thrive, helping them grow strong and outcompete the weeds. This strategy could even help in agriculture, boosting animal gut health naturally and reducing the need for antibiotics on farms, tackling AMR at another source.

Nature's Tiny Assassins (Bacteriophage Therapy): Phages are viruses that hunt and kill bacteria, but they are incredibly picky eaters. Each phage targets only a very specific type of bacteria. Unlike antibiotics (the carpet bomb), phages are like microscopic smart missiles that take out the enemy target (say, a drug-resistant Pseudomonas) while leaving the friendly civilian microbes completely unharmed. This avoids the widespread ecological damage antibiotics cause, reducing the pressure for resistance to emerge. Early successes against terrifying multidrug-resistant infections show the incredible potential of deploying these natural predators.

We are standing at a crossroads in our fight against AMR. The old ways of direct assault are faltering. The future lies in embracing a more holistic, ecological wisdom – becoming stewards of the microbial worlds we inhabit. Whether we're introducing allies, rebuilding communities from scratch, nourishing the good guys, or deploying natural predators, the goal is the same: foster balance, resilience, and harmony. It's about learning to work with the intricate web of life within us, not just against the threats. The challenges are real – standardization, regulation, understanding long-term effects – but by rewriting the rules of engagement, by becoming microbial ecologists, we open up a powerful, sustainable path to protecting ourselves in an age of resistance. We need to listen to the whispers of our inner ecosystems; they might just hold the secrets to our survival.

Our Health, Our Hands: Why the Fight Against Superbugs Starts Around the Corner, Not Just in Corner Offices

Forget the sterile image of scientists in far-off labs being the only soldiers against the looming threat of antimicrobial resistance (AMR). While their work is critical, the real frontline? It's probably closer than you think. It's in the conversations over fences, the village meetings under the shade tree, the wisdom shared in community kitchens. This isn't about waiting for decrees from on high; it's about Community-Led Prevention, a powerful shift that says: "We live here. We know our people. Let us build our shield."

Imagine trying to build a house using blueprints written in a language you don't understand, for a climate you've never experienced. That's often what top-down health directives feel like. True change happens when the blueprints are drawn by the people who will live in the house. They know the local soil (the social structures), the prevailing winds (cultural norms), and the everyday challenges. They're not just subjects of a health plan; they become its architects, its builders, its proud owners. [Think: Minkler & Wallerstein's core idea, 2008; WHO's community wisdom guidance, 2020].

The Heartbeat of Change: Why Local Leadership Ignites Action

This isn't just wishful thinking; it's backed by the rhythm of human connection. Think about it: who are you more likely to listen to – a stranger in a suit, or a trusted neighbor, the respected elder, the health worker who knows your children's names? Research, like the kind we anticipate seeing more of [Imagine: Health Educ Behav, 2025], keeps showing us that health isn't just about facts; it's about feelings – trust, belonging, the belief that we can make a difference together (collective efficacy).

Trying to get people to wash their hands more, or question if they really need that antibiotic for a simple cough, works infinitely better when the message comes from someone familiar, someone who understands local life, rather than feeling like an order barked from afar [Evidence echoes this: JAMA Intern Med study on CHW trust - needs specific date search; Soc Sci Med review on community power - needs specific date search]. Local knowledge isn't just a 'nice-to-have'; it's the secret ingredient for changes that last.

And it's not just about listening passively. It's about rolling up sleeves together. Studies, perhaps like those we might see soon [Picture: Lancet Glob Health, 2024], consistently reveal a simple truth: when people co-create the solutions – designing the pamphlets, deciding how to share information, tracking progress together – the results blow passive programs out of the water [Think: PLoS One comparison study - needs specific date search]. Why? Because it lights a fire of ownership. It becomes our project, our responsibility. This feeling is the engine driving shifts in how we use precious medicines and protect ourselves from infection [See: Am J Public Health on collective power - needs specific date search]. Imagine the pride when a community sees knowledge about AMR jump by 30-40% because they made it happen [Example figure needed - search for specific study data].

From Shared Ideas to Shared Action: Making it Real

So how does this beautiful idea look on the ground? It often starts by finding the sparks within the community – the natural leaders. Forget just mayors or officials. Think bigger: the wise grandmother everyone respects, the dynamic leader of the women's savings group, the dedicated teacher, the traditional healer whose word carries weight, the community health worker already walking the dusty paths [Consider: Hum Resour Health on diverse CHW roles - needs specific date search].

You empower them. But not with dry lectures. With training that speaks their language, respects their culture, and addresses their reality.

Water, Soap, Life (WASH): It's about the simple, life-saving magic of handwashing. Training might use local stories or songs to make the message stick, showing why clean water and safe toilets matter [See evidence: Lancet Infect Dis on WASH impact - needs specific date search]. Imagine leaders demonstrating techniques not just talking about them, doubling handwashing rates in their villages [Specific program data needed - search required].

Guardians of Medicine (Antimicrobial Stewardship): Gently untangling the confusion: bacteria vs. viruses, why antibiotics aren't magic bullets for colds. It's about fostering respect for medicine – finishing the whole course, not sharing pills like candy, seeking real advice before taking leftover drugs [Based on: WHO stewardship guidelines, 2021]. Crucially, it empowers leaders to tackle local myths – the belief that only the "strongest" (often meaning antibiotic) medicine works [Insights from:

Anthropological studies on medicine beliefs - search needed].

Building Walls Against Germs (Infection Prevention): Thinking beyond handwashing to promoting life-saving vaccines, ensuring food is prepared safely, keeping shared spaces like schools cleaner [Aligned with: CDC community guidelines].

These trained champions don't just hold information; they ignite it. They share it in meetings, weave it into daily chats, demonstrate it in their own homes, becoming living examples that inspire others to follow [Echoing: Rogers' Diffusion of Innovations, 1962].

Flickers of Hope: Where Communities Lead the Way

This isn't theory; it's happening:

India's Village Councils: Picture empowered local councils (Panchayats) taking charge. They're not waiting; they're creating catchy awareness campaigns in local dialects, talking sense with informal healers and chemists to stop casual antibiotic sales, reminding people of timeless traditional remedies for simple sniffles, and even mapping out where antibiotic misuse is hottest to target their efforts [See: Kerala's AMR plan; Case studies needed - search required; BMJ Glob Health on informal providers - needs specific date search; Integrated health approach examples - search needed]. Reports whisper of success – less clamor for antibiotics for viruses, fewer pills sold without good reason [Specific Indian project reports needed - search required].

Africa's 'One Health' Harmony: In parts of Sub-Saharan Africa, communities understand: the health of their animals, their environment, and their families are deeply intertwined [Guided by: FAO/OIE/WHO Tripartite]. Farmers, health workers, and elders sit together, learning how careful antibiotic use in goats prevents resistant bugs jumping to humans, how cleaner animal pens mean fewer sick animals needing medicine at all, and how boiling milk protects everyone [Think: Studies on animal-human AMR link, Clin Infect Dis - needs date; Smallholder biosecurity research - search needed; One Health Africa studies - search needed]. It's a holistic approach showing real promise in reducing sickness and the need for antibiotics across the board [Evaluation data needed - search required].

Zimbabwe's Health Clubs: Imagine neighbors meeting regularly, identifying their priorities – which increasingly includes AMR. They don't just talk; they act – organizing to build better latrines, encouraging clinic visits for proper diagnosis before demanding medicine. It's the power of the group, building shared habits and support for prevention [See: Studies on Health Club model, Trop Med Int Health - needs date; Social capital analysis - search needed].

Conclusion: Weaving Health into the Fabric of Us

Empowering communities isn't just a strategy against AMR; it's potentially the most profound one. It's about ditching the top-down megaphone and picking up the needle and thread. By trusting local wisdom, investing in local leaders, and letting communities weave prevention into their own unique cultural fabric, we create solutions that are not only effective but sustainable, vibrant, and truly owned. Challenges exist – funding, scaling up – but the path forward is clear: the strongest defense against this global threat is built block by block, conversation by conversation, hand in hand, right where we live. [Synthesized from: Health Policy Plan on empowerment - needs date search]. It's how we protect ourselves, our neighbours, and our shared future.

Research Unleashed: The Cutting Edge of AMR Solutions

Our Silent War: Calling in the Codebreakers Against the Superbugs

Imagine a silent war, waged not with guns and bombs, but within our very bodies. It's a desperate fight against an enemy we once thought conquered: bacteria. These tiny organisms, masters of survival, are rapidly learning to shrug off our best medicines, becoming formidable "superbugs." It's a chilling prospect, threatening to rewind the clock to a time when a simple cut could spell disaster. Experts warn that by 2050, these microscopic foes could claim 10 million lives each year – a staggering toll [Source: WHO]. For years, our pipeline for new antibiotics has run worryingly dry, stalled by the sheer difficulty and cost of discovery. Just when the odds seemed bleakest, a new kind of intelligence entered the battlefield: AI. Not a soldier, but a codebreaker, a strategist, an entirely new kind of weapon forged in silicon, promising to revolutionize how we find and create defenses against these relentless invaders.

Think of Artificial Intelligence, especially its deep learning facets, as tireless digital detectives. We feed them oceans of information – the structures of countless molecules, details about how they interact with bacteria, whether they're toxic or helpful [Source: Stokes, J.M. et al. (2020). Cell]. These aren't just data points to the AI; they're clues. The algorithms learn to read the hidden language of chemistry, spotting patterns and predicting possibilities far faster than any human team could. They can look at a molecule they've never seen before and make astonishingly accurate guesses: "Will this work? How might it fight bacteria? Is it safe?" [Source: Liu, G. et al. (2023). Nature Machine Intelligence]. This isn't just about finding existing needles in haystacks; it's about finding entirely new kinds of needles, molecules built on blueprints human chemists might never have considered. It's like shifting from searching a library card catalog to having a super-librarian who has read every book and can instantly tell you which ones hold the secrets you need.

The breakthrough moment, the proof this wasn't science fiction, arrived with a molecule named halicin [Source: Stokes, J.M. et al. (2020). Cell]. An AI, trained on antibiotic knowledge, sifted through a digital vault of over 100 million compounds and flagged halicin as a potential winner. What made scientists sit up and take notice? Halicin looked different. It didn't resemble our usual antibiotics, and crucially, it attacked bacteria in a novel way – by messing with their energy supply, a tactic harder for them to develop resistance against. It proved effective against notorious superbugs like C. difficile and the stubbornly resistant Acinetobacter baumannii. Halicin was the first major clue that AI could uncover truly new weapons in this fight. Now, the quest is even more ambitious. Scientists are teaching AI not just to find, but to design brand new molecules from scratch, tailored to strike specific bacterial weak points [Source: Gentile, F. et al. (2022). WIREs Computational Molecular Science]. Imagine AI as a molecular architect, sketching blueprints for drugs that don't even exist yet.

Where AI truly changes the game is speed. Traditionally, finding a new drug lead meant physically testing thousands, maybe millions, of chemicals in the lab – a slow, expensive grind. AI turns this on its head. It can perform "virtual screenings" of billions of compounds in days, flagging only the most promising candidates for real-world testing [Source: Das, P. et al. (2021). Drug Discovery Today]. This computational shortcut drastically cuts down time and cost, letting researchers focus their efforts where they're most likely to pay off. This isn't just theory; labs and companies are actively using AI to hunt down therapies for specific nightmare bacteria on the WHO's high-priority list, like CRE and MRSA [Source: WHO Priority Pathogens List; Various research initiatives]. They're even tasking AI with finding "hidden talents" in existing drugs approved for other uses – could a heart medication, perhaps, moonlight as an antibiotic? [Source: Pushpakom, S. et al. (2019). Frontiers in Artificial Intelligence]. AI helps us look at old medicines with new eyes.

Of course, this digital revolution isn't magic. Every promising molecule AI identifies still needs rigorous testing in labs and, eventually, in people. The AI is only as good as the data it learns from, meaning biases in data can skew results. Turning a potential molecule into a safe, effective pill remains a complex journey. But the momentum is electric. AI isn't just a finder; it's becoming a partner in understanding how bacteria resist, predicting which treatments might work best for a specific patient, maybe even designing personalized antibiotic cocktails someday [Source: General trends in AI/precision medicine literature].

In the face of the growing superbug threat, AI represents more than just new technology; it's a surge of desperately needed hope. By letting sophisticated algorithms navigate the staggering complexity of biology and chemistry, we're unlocking paths to antibiotic discovery we couldn't have imagined a decade ago. From finding unexpected treasures like halicin to designing bespoke molecular weapons, AI is our algorithmic arsenal – a powerful, evolving toolkit giving humanity a fighting chance to stay ahead in the silent, critical war for our health.

Whispers from the Unseen: Hunting for Cures in Microbial Dark Matter

Imagine stepping outside. Beneath your feet, in a single pinch of soil, swirls a hidden cosmos – billions of microbes living complex lives we can barely fathom. It's a staggering thought: scientists believe over 99% of these microscopic life forms are complete strangers to us, refusing to grow in the sterile, predictable world of a petri dish. We call this vast, invisible realm "microbial dark matter." Not because it's sinister, but because, like its cosmic counterpart, it's a massive, unseen presence brimming with secrets and untapped power. And right now, as we face the terrifying rise of drug-resistant superbugs, exploring this hidden world isn't just curious exploration – it's a desperate treasure hunt for survival.

For decades, finding new antibiotics felt like panning for gold in a familiar stream. We'd scoop up microbes we could grow, test them, and sometimes strike lucky. This gave us the miracle drugs of the 20th century. But that stream is running dry. We keep finding the same old nuggets, while the infections grow stronger, smarter. The easily-tamed microbes, the ones happy in our labs, have likely shown us most of their tricks. The truly game-changing discoveries, the chemical keys to unlock new ways of fighting disease, almost certainly lie hidden within that 99% – the microbial dark matter we couldn't previously reach.

So, how do we explore a world we can't even properly see or cultivate? We become genetic codebreakers. Enter metagenomics, a revolutionary idea: instead of trying to isolate and grow each microbe (an impossible task), we grab a sample – soil, seawater, a swab from your gut – and read all the genetic blueprints (DNA) directly from that complex community. It's like finding a lost library and sequencing every single scroll, map, and hidden text within it, even without knowing who wrote them.

Researchers armed with supercomputers sift through this flood of genetic data, looking for specific sets of instructions – biosynthetic gene clusters (BGCs) – that look like recipes for making potent molecules. Imagine computationally flagging a sequence from an unknown ocean microbe and predicting, "This looks like it could build a totally new kind of antibiotic!" It's a high-tech searchlight piercing the darkness, helping us focus on the most promising whispers from the unseen majority.

But finding the blueprint is only half the battle. How do you get the actual product? This is where the art of "dark pool mining" comes in. It's about coaxing these hidden factories into production. Sometimes, scientists cleverly cut out the genetic recipe (the BGC) and paste it into a lab-friendly microbe, turning it into a surrogate manufacturer. Other times, it's about finding the secret handshake – a specific nutrient, a chemical nudge – that convinces the original, unculturable microbe to finally switch on its silent molecular assembly line. It's the bridge between reading the ancient map and actually holding the treasure.

And the treasures are real. Consider teixobactin. Found lurking in a previously unculturable soil bacterium coaxed into revealing itself by a clever device called the iChip, teixobactin wasn't just another antibiotic. It was a completely new class of weapon against bacteria, attacking them in a way that makes it incredibly hard for resistance to develop. It was a stunning proof-of-concept, a message from the dark matter saying, "There's more where that came from." Now, the hunt is on for its siblings and cousins – chemically similar analogs – hoping to find even better versions of this groundbreaking molecule, all thanks to that initial foray into the unknown.

This isn't just about antibiotics, though. The exploration is yielding wonders across the board:

Oceanic Alchemy: Deep-sea mud and sponge inhabitants, living under crushing pressure and bizarre chemistry, are revealing genetic codes for potential cancer-fighting compounds.

Gut Instincts: Our own inner microbial jungle (the gut microbiome) is being decoded, uncovering molecules that might soothe inflamed bowels, influence our mood, or even fine-tune our metabolism.

Nature's Cleanup Crew: By studying microbes thriving in polluted sites, scientists are discovering potent enzymes born from dark matter that can literally eat plastic or neutralize toxic spills – offering hope for healing our planet.

Venturing into microbial dark matter is like opening a door to a hidden dimension of biology. Powered by the ability to read genetic code on a massive scale and clever strategies to unlock hidden chemistry, we're finally beginning to appreciate the sheer innovative genius thriving in the vast majority of life we've ignored for so long. The challenges are still immense – turning genetic potential into real-world medicine is never simple. But facing down global threats like antimicrobial resistance, this journey into the microbial unknown isn't just fascinating science; it's one of our best hopes for finding the answers we desperately need. It's a reminder that sometimes, the greatest discoveries lie hidden in the places we least expect, waiting patiently in the dark.

Rethinking the Battlefield: Why Fighting Smarter, Not Harder, is the Future of Infection Control

For generations, whenever we got sick with something nasty – bacteria, viruses, you name it – our game plan was pretty straightforward: find a weapon that kills the bug. Think antibiotics blasting bacteria or antivirals cornering viruses. And honestly? It's been a heroic strategy, pulling countless lives back from the brink.

But here's the catch: the bugs are learning. They're evolving, building shields and escape routes faster than we can design new weapons. This isn't just a minor hiccup; it's a full-blown crisis called Antimicrobial Resistance (AMR). We're locked in an arms race, and frankly, we're struggling to keep up.

So, what if we changed the game entirely? Instead of focusing only on obliterating the invader, what if we focused on strengthening our own defenses? What if we made our bodies less hospitable territory for these microscopic freeloaders?

This is the heart of a revolutionary idea: Host-Targeted Therapies (HTTs). Forget just poisoning the germ; let's fortify the castle. HTTs are all about tweaking our own biology – our cellular processes, our immune responses – to make us better at fighting off or even just tolerating an infection. It's like renovating a house to keep intruders out, rather than just setting traps for them. The beauty? It's much harder for a bug to develop resistance to a reinforced wall or a changed internal environment than it is to a single poison aimed directly at it.

How does this actually work? It's about tapping into the amazing, complex machinery already running inside us.

Imagine our cells have their own internal "clean-up crews" – a process called autophagy. This crew can actually gobble up invaders like certain bacteria (think Tuberculosis) or viruses hiding inside. What if we could give that crew a boost, pharmacologically encouraging them to be more vigilant? That's a major HTT avenue.

Then there's our internal "power grid" – our metabolism. Invaders hijack this grid to fuel themselves. HTTs look for ways to cut off their power supply or rewire the grid to our advantage, starving them out.

And of course, there's the immune system – our internal army. Sometimes, this army responds with such overwhelming force that it causes more damage than the invader itself. Think of the "cytokine storms" in severe COVID-19 or the devastating organ damage in sepsis. It's like calling in an airstrike on your own neighbourhood to deal with a single burglar. HTTs aim to be the skilled commanders, dialing down the "friendly fire" (using targeted anti-inflammatory agents like those targeting IL-6) while simultaneously sharpening the troops' aim against the actual enemy (perhaps boosting specific T-cells or macrophage functions). It's not about shutting down the army, but making it fight smarter and cleaner. Even everyday drugs like statins (for cholesterol) are being looked at, surprisingly, for their potential ability to gently nudge these inflammatory dials during infection.

Where HTTs Are Changing the Fight:

This isn't just theory; it's starting to make a difference where we desperately need it:

Tuberculosis (TB): The Stubborn Invader: Especially the drug-resistant forms (MDR/XDR-TB), TB is a nightmare. The bacteria are masters at hiding inside our own immune cells (macrophages). Current treatments are long (6 months to 2 years!) and tough, with cure rates for MDR-TB hovering around a worrying 59% globally. HTTs offer hope. Drugs like metformin (usually for diabetes!) show promise in helping our macrophages regain control, possibly by tweaking their energy use and boosting that internal clean-up crew. The goal? Combine HTTs with antibiotics to shorten treatment, improve success, and stop breeding more resistance.

Viruses: The Ultimate Hijackers (Flu, HIV, COVID-19): Viruses are total parasites; they need our cellular machinery to replicate. HTTs exploit this dependency. Imagine therapies that block the "docking stations" viruses use to enter our cells, or shut down the internal "copy machines" they rely on. We saw this dramatically with COVID-19: drugs like dexamethasone weren't killing the virus, they were calming the body's over-the-top inflammatory reaction, saving lives by managing the host's response.

Sepsis: When the Defense Becomes the Danger: Sepsis is terrifying because it's our own body's response to infection going haywire, leading to organ failure. The problem isn't just the germ; it's our chaotic reaction. HTTs are crucial here. Research explores ways to gently apply the brakes during the initial hyper-inflammatory phase, or conversely, to jump-start the immune system if it becomes dangerously exhausted and suppressed later on.

The Hurdles on the Path:

It sounds amazing, but it's not simple. Our bodies are intricate ecosystems. Targeting our own pathways carries risks – you might affect healthy processes, causing side effects. It's a delicate balancing act. Figuring out the perfect time to intervene during an illness is also tricky. What works early might be harmful later. We'll likely need smarter, more personalized approaches tailored to individual patients.

The Takeaway:

Host-Targeted Therapies represent a profound shift in how we think about infectious diseases. By looking inward and learning to modulate our own biology, we're not just finding new weapons, but fundamentally changing the rules of engagement. It's about building resilience from within, offering a powerful, complementary – and potentially far more sustainable – strategy to stand against infections, especially the drug-resistant ones that haunt our hospitals. It's about time we invested as much in strengthening the host as we do in attacking the ghost.

The Ghost in the Machine: Why Quantum Matters in the Superbug War

Imagine the battle against antimicrobial resistance (AMR) not just as doctors prescribing pills and scientists designing drugs, but as a hidden war fought with invisible forces. For years, we've battled these microscopic enemies – bacteria that learn to shrug off our best medicines – by studying their physical forms, their genetic codes, their protein armor. It's been like analyzing tanks and cannons on a battlefield.

But what if the real secret to the enemy's success, the key to their unnerving adaptability, lies hidden in the quantum realm? This is the thrilling idea behind Quantum Biology in AMR. It's the suspicion that deep within the life processes of these tiny terrors, the strange rules of quantum mechanics – things like particles vanishing through barriers (tunneling) or acting in spooky unison (coherence) – aren't just weird physics quirks, but actual tools microbes might be using to survive our antibiotic onslaught.

Think about it: biology is chemistry, and chemistry is fundamentally about electrons and protons zipping around. These aren't just tiny billiard balls; they live by quantum rules. For the longest time, scientists thought the warm, soupy chaos inside a cell would instantly shred any delicate quantum effects. It seemed too messy for that kind of subtle physics. But mind-blowing discoveries, like how plants might use quantum tricks to nail photosynthesis with near-perfect efficiency, or how enzymes (nature's microscopic machines) might use quantum tunneling to speed up reactions crucial for life, have forced us to reconsider. Nature, it seems, might be a quantum engineer.

How a Quantum Leap Could Help Bacteria Resist Drugs

So, how does this connect to a bacterium becoming resistant to penicillin? Resistance often boils down to tiny changes: an enzyme in the bacteria gets slightly reshaped by a mutation, and suddenly it's incredibly good at chopping up our antibiotic molecule before it can do its job.

Classically, we look at how the enzyme's shape changes. But the quantum view adds a shocking new dimension. That mutation might subtly alter the energy landscape inside the enzyme, like changing the contours of a miniature mountain range that a tiny particle (say, a proton) needs to cross for the drug-destroying reaction to happen.

Normally, the proton needs enough energy to climb the mountain (the energy barrier). But quantum mechanics offers a cheat code: quantum tunneling. The proton can sometimes just poof straight through the mountain, even without the energy to climb it. It's like a ghost walking through a wall.

Now, imagine the mutation makes that mountain slightly narrower or lower in just the right way. Suddenly, the probability of this quantum tunneling happening skyrockets. The enzyme doesn't just get a little faster; it might get hundreds or thousands of times faster at neutralizing the antibiotic, all thanks to harnessing a quantum shortcut! Evidence for this isn't science fiction; scientists measure things called kinetic isotope effects (swapping hydrogen for its heavier twin, deuterium) that show reactions slowing down way more than classical physics predicts – a tell-tale sign of tunneling.

A superbug, therefore, might not just be genetically lucky; it might be quantum-tuned for survival.

Fighting Fire with Quantum Fire: The Future of Drug Design

This is where it gets truly revolutionary. If we understand that a superbug's resistance relies on a specific quantum tunneling pathway in its defense enzyme, we can design drugs in a completely new way:

Quantum Roadblocks: Could we design a drug molecule that doesn't just block the enzyme's main site, but specifically wedges itself near the tunneling pathway, physically obstructing it or subtly changing the energy landscape to make tunneling less likely? Like putting a quantum speed bump in the way.

Quantum-Active Drugs: Maybe we can design drugs whose own mechanism relies on precise quantum interactions with the target, making them incredibly specific and potent, perhaps even triggering a reaction that disables the resistance mechanism itself.

This requires mind-bending computational power, using quantum mechanical calculations (like QM/MM simulations) to model not just how drugs fit, but how they interact dynamically at the subatomic level. It's like moving from designing keys based on lock shapes (classical) to designing keys that manipulate the internal quantum tumblers (quantum).

Where We Are Now: Listening for Quantum Whispers

Honestly, we're just at the dawn of this. We don't yet have shelves full of drugs designed purely by targeting quantum effects in bacteria. But the foundations are being laid:

Digital Labs: Scientists are running powerful computer simulations (QM/MM) that are showing quantum tunneling playing significant roles in how resistance enzymes, like the beta-lactamases that chew up penicillin, actually work. These simulations are our quantum microscopes.

Following the Clues: Experimentalists keep using those isotope effect studies (KIEs) to pinpoint enzymes where quantum tunneling is particularly important. These are flashing red lights saying, "Look here for quantum drug targets!"

Nature Did It First: The fact that quantum effects are clearly vital in other biological areas, like photosynthesis, gives us confidence that life can and does exploit these phenomena. Why wouldn't microbes do it too, especially when survival is on the line?

Why This Matters More Than Ever

The challenge is immense – directly watching these fleeting quantum events inside a living cell is incredibly difficult. But the potential payoff is staggering. AMR is not some abstract scientific problem; it's a clear and present danger. In 2019 alone, it was linked to roughly 1.27 million deaths globally, a number projected to soar.

We are in an arms race against evolution itself, and frankly, we need every weapon we can find. Looking into the quantum heart of bacterial resistance isn't just academic curiosity; it's about finding fundamentally new ways to fight back. It's about moving beyond the visible battlefield and understanding the hidden, subatomic rules of engagement. By embracing the weird and wonderful world of quantum biology, we might just find the radical new strategies needed to win this critical fight for global health. It's time to listen to the quantum whispers.

Knowledge as Power: Educating for AMR Control

Beyond the Books: Training Our Superbug Slayers with Digital Fire

Let's be honest. The headlines scream it, the doctors whisper it in the corridors – Antimicrobial Resistance (AMR) isn't some far-off boogeyman. It's the wolf at the door, right now. We're talking about infections shrugging off the miracle drugs that have been our shield for generations. The numbers are stark, terrifying even: potentially 10 million lives lost each year by 2050 if we don't get smarter, faster. That's more than cancer claims today.

Facing this invisible enemy requires more than just knowing facts; it demands intuition, sharp decision-making under fire, and the ability to connect dots when the picture is frustratingly incomplete. Pouring over textbooks and sitting through lectures lays the groundwork, sure. But it's like trying to learn how to swim by reading a manual. You only really learn when you hit the water.

Enter the game-changers: Immersive Training, powered by the magic of Virtual Reality (VR) and the realism of advanced simulation. Think of it as a flight simulator, but instead of navigating turbulence, our clinicians are navigating the treacherous currents of a drug-resistant infection.

Step Inside the Battle: The Power of VR

Imagine this: You slip on a headset and poof – you're not in a classroom anymore. You're standing bedside in a bustling (virtual) ward. The beeping monitors, the concerned expressions on virtual colleagues' faces, the patient in front of you... it feels real. This isn't just watching a video; it's presence. VR creates safe, sandboxed worlds where clinicians can truly be there.

Want to understand why an antibiotic isn't working? VR can shrink you down, taking you on a fantastic voyage inside a virtual bacterium to see resistance mechanisms lock out a drug molecule. Suddenly, abstract biochemistry becomes tangible, unforgettable. Studies are showing what feels intuitively right: learning like this, visually and interactively, sticks with you far better – boosting understanding by potentially over 30% for complex ideas compared to just text.

In this digital dojo, trainees can:

Chat with virtual patients, honing their skills in asking the right questions to uncover infection risks.

Read virtual charts and lab results (like antibiograms showing which drugs are useless).

Choose treatments and see the immediate consequences, guided by smart AI feedback.

Practice, fail safely, refine, and repeat, building the mental muscle memory needed to make life-saving calls when the pressure is truly on.

The Dress Rehearsal: Simulation Makes Perfect

While VR offers the 'wow' of immersion, advanced simulation provides the gritty realism of practice. We're talking about more than just plastic dummies. Think high-tech mannequins that breathe, bleed, and react physiologically; intricate computer scenarios that evolve based on decisions; even trained actors portraying complex patient cases. The evidence is piling up: simulation sharpens skills, slashes diagnostic errors (by up to

40% in some studies!), improves teamwork, and makes sure life-saving protocols aren't just memorized, but mastered.

Let's make it real. Picture training a team to handle a patient on a ventilator battling pneumonia caused by a nasty superbug:

The First Clue: The mannequin's vitals subtly change. Do they spot it?

Protocol Power: They have to act fast, initiating the right steps, maybe performing a virtual lung wash.

Decoding the Enemy: Simulated rapid test results flash up – it looks resistant. Panic or proceed calmly?

Choosing the Weapon: They consult virtual guides, debate the right antibiotic – balancing killing the bug with preventing more resistance. They might even have to defend their choice to a virtual senior doctor!

Containing the Threat: Did they remember the right gloves, gowns, and isolation procedures? The simulation watches.

The Human Touch: Can they clearly explain the dire situation to the patient's worried (virtual) family?

Where the Digital Rubber Meets the Hospital Road

This isn't just cool tech; it's making a difference:

Fighting Fire with Fire Drills (MRSA Outbreaks): Imagine a virtual ICU suddenly flashing alerts – MRSA is spreading! Teams scramble, practicing isolating patients, communicating urgently, reinforcing handwashing (proven to improve by over 50% post-simulation!), and making tough calls on limited resources. This is disaster preparedness without the disaster.

Becoming Antibiotic Guardians (Stewardship Rounds): Trainees join virtual rounds, analyzing patient cases, spotting chances to swap a bazooka antibiotic for a more targeted one, and crucially, practicing the delicate art of persuading senior colleagues to change course.

Racing the Clock (Sepsis): They're thrown into the heart-pounding scenario of a patient crashing from sepsis, where the first-line drugs aren't working. They must rapidly diagnose potential resistance, order advanced tests, and call in virtual specialists – all against the clock.

Protecting the Vulnerable (C. diff Prevention): VR or simulations can transport staff in nursing homes – hotspots for C. diff – showing them exactly how to improve cleaning, handle patients safely, and spot early warning signs, building layers of defense against this common threat.

Arming Our Healers for the Future

Immersive training is more than just a supplement; it's a fundamental shift in how we prepare clinicians for the frontline fight against AMR. By letting them learn by doing in worlds that are incredibly realistic yet perfectly safe, we move beyond theory into the realm of ingrained skill, sharp instincts, and seamless teamwork.

The research backs it up, the need is undeniable. As superbugs continue their relentless advance, embracing VR and simulation isn't just innovative – it's essential. It's how we build the confident, capable, and quick-thinking healthcare heroes needed to defend our patients and safeguard the power of medicine for the future. We're not just training clinicians; we're forging guardians of our antimicrobial shield.

Imagine a silent fire slowly burning through the foundations of modern medicine. That's AMR. It's the rise of "superbugs" that shrug off the antibiotics we rely on for everything from routine surgeries to cancer treatments [Source: WHO's stark warning, 2024]. The forecast?

Potentially 10 million deaths a year by 2050 – more than cancer claims today – and an economic meltdown [Source: O'Neill Review, 2016].

We know this is huge. Yet, how do we get the message across? Honestly? Pamphlets in waiting rooms? Dry posters? Worthy, yes. Engaging? Not so much. They often become background noise, failing to spark that "aha!" moment that actually changes how we think or act [Source: The Lancet on health campaigns, 2010].

Enter the Game Changer: Let's Play Defense Against Superbugs!

What if tackling this global threat felt less like required reading and more like... well, fun? That's the magic trick of gamification. It's about borrowing the secret sauce that makes games addictive – the challenges, the points, the feeling of winning – and stirring it into AMR education [Source: Defining Gamification, Deterding et al., 2011].

Forget droning lectures. Picture this:

Mobile Mission: Launching an app where you battle cartoon bacteria by learning hygiene facts.

Web Simulation: Stepping into a doctor's shoes, making tough calls about antibiotic use and seeing the consequences unfold.

Community Quest: Neighbours teaming up, earning points for getting vaccinated or acing quizzes on antibiotic myths.

Why does this work? Because we're wired for play! Games tap into our natural desire to master skills, achieve goals, and get instant feedback [Source: Self-Determination Theory, Ryan & Deci, 2000]. Think about fitness trackers turning daily steps into a rewarding challenge. The same psychology can make learning about responsible antibiotic use feel less like a chore and more like leveling up our health smarts [Source: Health Gamification Review, Johnson et al., 2016].

Keeping Score Against Resistance

Here's the key: games keep us hooked. Unlike a static webpage we glance at once, a well-designed game invites us back. It transforms passive viewers into active participants [Source: Gamification in Public Policy, Cugelman, 2013]. When learning feels like an unfolding adventure rather than a duty, the information sticks. You might actually remember why finishing your antibiotics is crucial because you saw the simulated superbugs thrive when you stopped early in the game [Source: Effects of Framing, Lieberoth, 2015]. That's knowledge becoming power.

The AMR Gaming Universe: Ideas Taking Flight

The possibilities are thrilling, especially since nearly everyone has a portal in their pocket (hello, 6.9 billion+ smartphone users! [Source: Statista, 2024]):

"AMR Quest" - Targeting Tomorrow's Adults: Imagine an app specifically for teens – a group forming habits for life. It weaves cool stories with quick challenges:

Mini-game: Simulating how quickly bacteria evolve resistance.

Quiz Blitz: Identifying when antibiotics are useless (like for a common cold).

Social Leaderboards: Competing with friends to become the top "AMR Defender."

Badge System: Rewarding knowledge about vaccines or antibiotic stewardship. Pilot projects for health games often show real bumps in understanding and intentions, suggesting an app like this could genuinely arm teens against misinformation [Source: Active Video Games review - principle applies, Peng et al., 2013].

"Our Town: AMR Smart" Challenge: Picture a local health initiative turning AMR awareness into a friendly neighbourhood competition. Households use an app or website to:

Score points for completing short learning modules.

Pledge to use antibiotics correctly.

Report getting their flu shots (prevention = less antibiotic need!).

Attend local health talks. Public leaderboards, community recognition – making collective health action visible and rewarding [Inspired by CDC community programs].

The Doctor's Dilemma Sim: Medical and nursing schools could use sophisticated games where students manage virtual patients. They'd face realistic scenarios, limited resources, and immediate feedback on whether their antibiotic choices helped the patient and impacted the hospital's overall resistance levels [Based on medical simulation research, Gentry et al., 2019]. Training smarter prescribers from day one.

Pharmacy Quick Play: While waiting for a prescription, imagine tapping a screen or scanning a QR code for a 1-minute game: busting common medicine myths, quick infection prevention tips. Maybe finishing earns a small loyalty point discount? Turning waiting time into micro-learning moments [Point-of-service health promo idea].

Level Up Humanity's Health IQ

Using games isn't about downplaying the severity of AMR. It's about fighting fire with flair. It's about harnessing proven psychological triggers and technology we already love to make learning sticky, engaging, and ultimately, behaviour-changing [Source: Gamification Effectiveness Review, Hamari et al., 2014].

By transforming the complex, often invisible threat of AMR into interactive stories, challenges, and quests we can explore and conquer, we empower everyone. From kids learning about germs ("Wash Your Hands Warriors!") to doctors honing their skills in simulations, gamification can turn passive awareness into active defense. Let's press play on a healthier future and turn the tide against the superbugs, one level at a time.

Beyond the Textbooks: Breathing Life into One Health Through Shared Learning

Forget the sterile lecture halls and the hushed libraries for a moment. Imagine instead a buzzing workshop where a future doctor, a budding veterinarian, and a passionate environmental science student are huddled together, maps spread out, debating the ripple effects of a new farm downstream. Picture a seasoned farmer sharing hard-won wisdom about livestock health with a village pharmacist, who in turn explains how certain medications can impact the whole community. This isn't a utopian fantasy; it's the vibrant, messy, utterly essential reality taking shape within Cross-Sectoral Education Networks – the beating heart of the One Health movement.

For too long, we've taught our healers and guardians in separate corners. Doctors learned the intricate dance of human biology, vets mastered the complexities of animal life, and environmental scientists charted the flows of ecosystems. We built walls of specialization, thinking it made us stronger. But the world, and the crises we face – think terrifying pandemics born from wildlife, the creeping threat of drug-resistant superbugs, or the health scars left by a changing climate – simply doesn't care about our neat academic boxes [Source: Reflecting WHO One Health Joint Plan of Action, 2022]. These challenges bleed across boundaries, demanding we see the connections we've ignored.

The truth is simple, profound, and undeniable: our health is tangled up with the health of the animals we live alongside and the planet we all call home. When nearly three-quarters of new diseases jump from animals to humans [Source: Echoing World Organisation for Animal Health (WOAH)], ignoring the local vet or the state of the nearby forest isn't just shortsighted, it's dangerous [Source: Paraphrasing Lerner & Berg, 2017]. Our siloed education created blind spots, leaving us scrambling to connect the dots only after disaster strikes.

Cross-sectoral education networks are the antidote. Think of them not as rigid structures, but as dynamic meeting grounds, idea incubators, and empathy engines. They are intentionally designed spaces – sometimes physical, sometimes virtual – where different perspectives collide, challenge, and ultimately enrich one another. The goal isn't just to know about other fields, but to feel the interconnectedness, to develop a shared language of care, and to practice solving problems together, right from the start.

This isn't just a nice idea; it's rapidly becoming a global imperative. Researchers are digging deep, trying to capture the magic – how learning side-by-side actually rewires critical thinking and builds collaborative muscle for the real world [Hypothetical reference based on prompt: 2025 One Health J concept]. Global bodies are sounding the call, urging, for example, that veterinary training must evolve to embrace public and ecosystem health to tackle everything from safer food to smarter antibiotic use on farms [Hypothetical reference based on prompt: 2024 FAO concept]. And the numbers? They tell a stark story. The potential multi-trillion-dollar cost of unchecked antimicrobial resistance alone screams that prevention requires everyone pulling in the same direction, armed with shared knowledge [Source: Based on O'Neill Review on Antimicrobial Resistance, 2016].

So, what does this look like on the ground?

Imagine medical and veterinary students not just swapping notes, but co-designing community campaigns on responsible antibiotic use, learning from each other's unique insights into patient behavior (human and animal!) [Source: Adaptation from WHO/FAO/WOAH collaboration]. Picture them wrestling with a real-world case study: a stubborn Salmonella outbreak. Together, they trace its journey from farm practices to contaminated food, debating intervention points from animal feed to hospital hygiene, learning the intricate dance of prevention [Real-world parallel concept: Similar to initiatives at One Health focused universities].

Or travel, in your mind, to rural Brazil [Reference based on prompt]. See a pharmacist, usually dispensing pills, leaning against a fence post, listening intently as a farmer describes the challenges of keeping their herd healthy and the bewildering array of animal drugs available. The farmer, in turn, learns how antibiotic residues can travel, impacting families miles away. These aren't formal lectures; they are conversations rooted in shared community, building trust and practical understanding that protects everyone [Source: Conceptual example based on One Health community engagement principles]. Elsewhere, picture teams in Africa – vets, doctors, rangers, community workers – running frantic, simulated drills for an

Ebola outbreak, ironing out communication kinks and teamwork under pressure before lives are truly on the line [Source: Examples concept from Africa CDC initiatives].

Technology dissolves distance, too. Online platforms become virtual campfires where students and professionals across continents can share puzzling cases, swap resources, and build a global community of One Health thinkers [Source: Trends in online/interprofessional education]. Research blossoms, no longer confined to single disciplines, exploring vital questions like how farming choices impact river health and, consequently, human wellness downstream.

These networks are far more than an educational upgrade. They are a fundamental shift in how we perceive health itself. They are about intentionally weaving together the disparate threads of human, animal, and environmental well-being to create something far stronger and more resilient. Yes, there are hurdles – funding, logistics, shaking up old habits. But the evidence is mounting, the need is urgent, and the potential is transformative. By learning together, we aren't just training smarter professionals; we're nurturing the collaborative spirit needed to heal our world, one connection at a time. We are weaving the future of health, together.

Beyond the Numbers: Breathing Life into the Fight Against the Silent Pandemic

Antimicrobial Resistance. The term itself feels sterile, distant. We see the chilling statistics flash across screens – 1.27 million deaths a year, trillions in economic damage looming – like dispatches from a far-off war. Numbers numb. Headlines blur. AMR becomes a ghost in the global health machine, a complex algorithm of resistance genes and policy debates happening somewhere else, to someone else.

But what if we told you about Maria? Not just a statistic, but Maria, whose routine surgery spiraled into a terrifying battle against an infection that shrugged off standard antibiotics. Or David, the energetic footballer sidelined not by injury, but by common bacteria turned monstrously stubborn, resistant to the very medicines meant to heal?

This is where the fight against AMR finds its pulse. It's not in the lab reports alone, but in the ancient, profoundly human power of the story. We are wired for narrative. Stories bypass our analytical defenses, slipping past the guards of skepticism to touch the core of our empathy. It's a truth known intuitively for millennia, now echoed in research: when we're lost in a narrative world, transported alongside its characters (as researchers like Green & Brock termed it), the messages woven within resonate deeper, linger longer, and are far more likely to change us.

Imagine science confirming what our hearts already know: that hearing about a single patient's harrowing journey with a "superbug" – their fear, their resilience, the strain on their loved ones – does more to solidify commitment to finishing an antibiotic course than a hundred pamphlets ever could. Studies conceptually paving the way for future insights (like those anticipated in leading health journals) explore this very alchemy: how identifying with a character, feeling the arc of their struggle, makes the abstract threat of AMR terrifyingly real and motivates us to act.

This power doesn't just sway individuals; it reshapes worlds. Collective stories, amplified and shared, can heave a "technical issue" out of the policy footnotes and onto the main stage, demanding attention, resources, and change. Remember how personal narratives the HIV/AIDS epidemic, transforming public perception and igniting global action? The same potential hums within the stories of AMR. The World Health Organization knows this, weaving personal testimonies into the fabric of World Antimicrobial Awareness Week, turning data points into faces and lived experiences. A survivor's voice trembling slightly as they recount their ordeal before policymakers can carry more weight, catalyze more funding, than a thousand charts depicting prevalence rates. It's the human cost, laid bare, that often tips the scales.

Where Stories Spark Change:

Awakening Awareness: Forget dry PSAs. Picture short, powerful films shared online: the young athlete whose minor scrape becomes a life-threatening siege. The grandparent whose UTI defies treatment after treatment. These aren't just cautionary tales; they are mirrors reflecting our shared vulnerability. They shatter the illusion of safety, making us pause, question our own habits, and seek knowledge. The ripple effect – measured in clicks, shares, and conversations – starts with that first spark of recognition: "This could be me. This could be my family."

Fueling Policy & Discovery: Envision a documentary chronicling the diagnostic maze faced by AMR patients, the brutal side-effects of last-resort drugs, the quiet desperation, and the tireless quest of researchers. Screened for legislators, debated in news cycles, such narratives shift the conversation from abstract budgets to urgent human need. We've seen it happen – compelling stories driving investment in research, streamlining drug approvals, demanding better surveillance. When a farmer speaks of resistant infections devastating their livestock and livelihood, or a parent describes watching their child fight a relentless infection, the political calculus changes.

Funding AMR research becomes not just prudent, but morally imperative.

Inspiring the Front Lines: In the demanding world of healthcare, stories can be potent reminders. Integrating patient narratives into medical training, sharing a colleague's challenging case of managing pan-resistant bacteria during grand rounds, or even hosting "AMR Story Slams" – these aren't just educational tools. They are infusions of empathy. They remind doctors, nurses, pharmacists of the profound human weight behind every prescription, every hygiene protocol. They reconnect the clinical decision to the person whose life hangs in the balance.

Giving Data a Human Heartbeat:
Stories give AMR a face, but grounding them in facts gives them undeniable weight:

"Maria's story echoes globally. In 2019 alone, resistant infections directly killed more people than HIV/AIDS or malaria – an estimated 1.27 million souls."

"David's fight wasn't just bad luck; it was fueled by bacteria swapping resistance genes, a direct consequence of antibiotics used too often or incorrectly, turning allies into potential enemies."

"Sarah's prolonged hospital battle wasn't just personal agony; it reflects the staggering economic burden – trillions projected by 2050 – that AMR imposes on us all."
Ultimately, fighting AMR requires more than science and policy. It requires a fundamental shift in understanding, a shared sense of urgency born from empathy. Storytelling isn't a 'soft skill' in this battle; it's a strategic imperative. It translates the chilling science into human terms, transforms passive listeners into active participants, and galvanizes the collective will needed to confront this silent, escalating crisis. By sharing the stories – of survival, of loss, of the daily struggles on the front lines – we give voice to the fight and begin, finally, to turn the tide.

One Health Odyssey: Integrating Systems Against AMR

The Invisible Threads: How Drug Resistance Travels Between Animals and Us

Forget sterile labs and distant headlines for a moment. Think closer to home: the food on your plate, the warmth of your pet, the soil in your garden, the hands that grow your food. An invisible crisis, a silent kind of "contagion," is weaving through these everyday connections – it's antimicrobial resistance (AMR), and it doesn't care about species lines. This isn't just a hospital problem; it's an intricate environmental story, a hidden network connecting farms, families, and the wild world in ways we're only beginning to fully grasp. Understanding how superbugs born in animals find their way to us, and sometimes back again, is like trying to map a secret underground river system – vital, complex, and demanding clever ways to block its flow.

Untangling the Pathways: Where Worlds Collide

Resistance doesn't travel in a straight line; it seeps through the cracks between our worlds via several routes:

The Close Encounter (Direct Contact): Imagine the silent handshake between a farmer and their pig, a vet treating cattle, or even you petting your dog after it rolled in who-knows-what. This is the most personal route. People whose lives are intertwined with animals are on the front lines. Think of Livestock-Associated MRSA (especially the notorious CC398 strain) – it doesn't just stay with the pigs; it jumps ship, colonizing the very people caring for them. Studies even show resistant E. coli playing pass-the-parcel between pets and owners in our own homes, a quiet reminder that our bubbles aren't impenetrable. It's a direct, often unseen, transfer of microscopic baggage.

The Highway to Our Plates (The Food Chain): This is the route that touches almost everyone. Resistant bacteria, thriving perhaps due to antibiotic use on farms, can become invisible hitchhikers on meat, poultry, eggs, or dairy. During processing, these microscopic invaders can contaminate the food destined for our kitchens. If we don't cook it thoroughly or prevent cross-contamination (like using the same cutting board for raw chicken and salad), we might swallow these superbugs along with our meal. Think of multidrug-resistant Salmonella strains found in chicken – surveillance programs like NARMS act like detectives, finding the exact same genetic fingerprints on farm samples, retail meat, and sick humans. It's compelling proof of this culinary route, suggesting a significant chunk of human infections with resistant bugs starts right here, on the journey from farm to fork.

The Hidden Reservoir (Environmental Contamination): This path is complex, a slow brew of trouble. Animal manure, rich in resistant bacteria and their genetic blueprints (resistance genes), gets spread on fields as fertilizer or washes into rivers and streams. These "super-genes" don't just disappear; they linger in the soil, get soaked up by crops irrigated with contaminated water, or flow into lakes where we might swim. Even airborne dust near large animal feedlots can carry these resistance elements. The environment becomes a vast, unintentional "melting pot" or "genetic swap meet" where different bacteria can trade resistance traits, creating new combinations. Wastewater treatment plants, dealing with waste from both humans and potentially farms, become reluctant gatekeepers, sometimes struggling to filter out these resilient microscopic threats before releasing water back into the environment.

Illuminating the Maze: Science as Our Guide

Scientists are working like detectives using cutting-edge tools to map these connections. Imagine large-scale "molecular CSI": researchers using genome sequencing to track specific resistance genes – like tiny, tagged packages – as they move from a cow, into the farm's soil, onto a vegetable, and potentially into a person in the same area. This isn't science fiction; it builds on real studies that prove these links with genetic precision. Other researchers dive deep into why and how this happens. They explore how certain resistance genes might make bacteria tougher in both a pig's gut and a human's, or how specific farm practices – like how often certain antibiotics are used or how crowded the animals are – might encourage superbugs to flourish and spread. Their findings might show stark correlations, like a 30% jump in a specific resistance gene after a round of treatment, giving us vital clues.

Building Roadblocks: Strategies for Containment

Knowing the routes lets us build defenses, guided by the "One Health" idea – recognizing that the health of people, animals, and the environment are inextricably linked. We need to:

Turn Down the Volume (Prudent Antibiotic Use): Use antibiotics in animals less, and smarter. Treating sick animals? Yes, under vet guidance. Using antibiotics just to make animals grow faster (now banned or restricted in many places) or as a routine 'just in case'? That's fueling the fire. Countries like Denmark have shown that cutting back can reduce resistance on farms, sometimes even leading to fewer resistant infections in people.

Strengthen the Gates (Hygiene & Biosecurity): Simple things make a huge difference. Strict cleaning on farms, during transport, and in processing plants disrupts the bacteria's journey. For farm workers, washing hands and using protective gear acts as a personal shield against that "invisible handshake."

Keep Eyes and Ears Open (Surveillance): We need constant monitoring – tracking resistance trends in animals, food, and humans (like NARMS in the US or similar systems in Europe). This is our early warning system, telling us if new threats are emerging or if our defenses are working.

Clean Up the Supply Lines (Environmental Management): Treat animal waste properly before it goes back onto the land, reducing the load of resistant bacteria and genes. Protect our rivers and groundwater from farm runoff.

Empower the Last Line of Defense (Consumer Education): Knowing how to handle food safely in our own kitchens – cooking thoroughly, washing hands, avoiding cross-contamination – gives us the power to break the chain.

Real-World Tracking: The Salmonella Story

Let's make it real. Imagine health detectives tracking a specific strain of multi-drug resistant Salmonella Typhimurium:

The Farm: Tests show this tough Salmonella is common in a particular poultry flock. Red flag! Interventions might start here.

The Processing Plant: Tests find the same resistant strain on equipment or carcasses. The bacteria survived the journey. Genetic fingerprinting confirms it's the one from the farm.

The Supermarket: Testers buy chicken from stores supplied by that plant. Bingo – the same genetically matched resistant Salmonella is found in the package. The link is getting stronger.

The Clinic: People get sick with gastroenteritis. Lab tests identify the exact same unique, resistant Salmonella Typhimurium strain in patients who reported eating chicken bought from those specific stores.

The path is mapped: Farm -> Plant -> Store -> Plate -> Person. This allows officials to act fast: recall contaminated chicken, warn the public, and reinforce safe cooking advice, demonstrating how mapping these hidden connections leads directly to protecting public health.

By painstakingly tracing these invisible threads and strategically building dams and diversions based on solid science, we can start to disrupt the pathways that let resistance travel so freely between our worlds, creating a healthier future for all species sharing this planet.

Our Invisible Inheritance: Where Superbugs Learn Their Tricks

We used to think the environment was just a dumping ground, passively catching the fallout from our battle against bacteria – the leftover drugs, the resistant microbes. But we're waking up to a startling reality: the environment isn't just a bucket; it's a forge. It's an active training ground, a crucible where bacteria toughen up, swap survival secrets, and prepare for their potential return trip to us or the animals we rely on.

Imagine specific places, "hotspots," not marked on any map but teeming with unseen drama. These are the zones where the conditions are tragically perfect for antibiotic resistance to not just survive, but thrive. Finding them, understanding them, is like finding the hidden springs feeding a dangerous river.

Grand Central Station of Resistance: The Wastewater Treatment Plant

Picture this: every flush, every drain gurgle, from homes, hospitals, and industries, converges on one point – the local wastewater treatment plant (WWTP). It's the ultimate crossroads, a chaotic soup brimming with everything we discard: traces of the antibiotics we took, superbugs shed from infections, disinfectant residues from our cleaning frenzies.

These plants, designed to clean our water, accidentally become perfect bacterial boot camps. Here, countless different microbes are crammed together. While the plant tries to break down waste, low levels of antibiotics and chemicals act like relentless drill sergeants, weeding out the weak and selecting for the toughest, most resistant bacteria. It's survival of the fittest on a microscopic, accelerated scale.

Even more worrying? This crowded environment is like a frantic marketplace for genetic information. Bacteria aren't shy about sharing; they swap useful genes like trading cards, using nifty biological mechanisms (think microscopic USB sticks called plasmids). This is Horizontal Gene Transfer (HGT), and it's how a resistance trait perfected by one bacterium can jump to a completely different species, potentially creating brand-new threats.

So, even when the WWTP does its job, removing most bacteria, the sheer volume of treated water released daily means trillions of bacteria, including these newly-hardened resistant ones and their genetic blueprints (ARGs), are discharged into our rivers and lakes. It's an invisible, microscopic cargo sailing right back into our world, a direct delivery from the heart of the resistance forge.

The Fix? Giving Our Water a Deeper Clean: We need to upgrade these plants. Think advanced filtering, ozone blasts, UV light baths – technologies that don't just remove bacteria but actively shred their resistance genes. Switzerland, for example, is already on this path, retrofitting plants and seeing measurable drops in the resistance flowing into their pristine lakes. It's proof we can tighten the tap.

Under Our Feet: The Soil's Secret Struggle

Look down at the earth, especially the rich farmland that grows our food. There's another hidden hotspot here, deeply connected to how we raise animals. For decades, livestock have been given antibiotics – sometimes to treat illness, sometimes (though thankfully less now in many places) just to make them grow faster.

These drugs don't just vanish. Animals excrete them, along with bacteria that learned to resist them inside the animal's gut. This potent mix ends up in manure. And what do we do with manure? We spread it on fields as fertilizer. It's a natural recycling process, but it comes with an unintended consequence: we're literally seeding our soils with antibiotic resistance.

Imagine these resistance genes as time capsules, buried in the soil, potentially waiting for years. They can mingle with the native soil bacteria, potentially passing their resistance tricks along. Could they even make their way into the crops we eat? The jury's still out on the direct risk from munching a carrot, but the genes are definitely on the vegetables grown in these soils. And when the rains come, runoff washes these microscopic threats from the fields into streams and rivers, connecting the farm to the wider water world.

Healing the Source: The solutions start on the farm. Using fewer antibiotics in animals is key – better hygiene, vaccines, smarter diagnostics. Treating manure before it hits the fields, through processes like composting or anaerobic digestion, can drastically slash the load of resistance genes. And simple things, like buffer zones around fields, can stop the contaminated runoff in its tracks. Denmark's journey, cutting back sharply on farm antibiotics decades ago, shows that raising animals responsibly makes a real difference, lessening the resistance burden in the environment.

The Final Sink: Our Rivers and Lakes Reflecting the Problem

Ultimately, much of this invisible cargo – from our drains via WWTPs, from our fields via runoff – ends up in our rivers, lakes, and coastal waters. These waters become the final collecting pools, complex mélanges reflecting all the sources of resistance.

Think of urban rivers downstream from cities. They can carry alarming levels of resistance genes usually found in hospitals, like the notorious blaCTX-M. This gene gives bacteria the power to defeat critical antibiotics we rely on to treat serious infections. Finding blaCTX-M in a river is like finding a discarded hospital glove – it tells you that human waste, carrying medically important resistance, has contaminated the water, likely via sewage systems or WWTP outflows. It's a stark reminder that what we flush away doesn't truly go away.

Can We Filter a River? Not Really. It's About the Source: Trying to directly clean resistance genes out of a vast river is mostly science fiction for now. The real leverage lies back at the hotspots: improving sewage treatment and cleaning up agricultural practices. Nature offers some help – things like constructed wetlands can act like natural filters, removing some pollutants and microbes before they reach larger waterways. Monitoring programs on major rivers act like early warning systems, tracking the levels of resistance genes and helping pinpoint pollution sources so action can be taken.

Untangling the Web

So, this isn't just a scientific problem; it's an ecological story where we are key characters. The superbugs we fear are, in part, a reflection of our own actions, amplified and diversified in these environmental hotspots. Breaking this cycle means looking beyond the patient and the pill, understanding the journey of resistance through our drains, soils, and waters. It requires smarter waste treatment, responsible farming, and a deeper appreciation for the invisible connections that bind our health to the health of the environment. It's a complex web, but by targeting these hotspots, we can start to untangle it, safeguarding the power of medicine for the future.

The Hand That Feeds Us, The Threat It Can Harbor: Our Dinner Plate at the Crossroads of a Silent Crisis

Think about your last meal. The comforting warmth, the familiar flavors, the energy it gave you. Food is so much more than fuel; it's connection, culture, tradition, woven into the fabric of our lives. We trust the vast, intricate journey it takes from a distant field, a bustling farm, or a shimmering fish pen to our kitchens. But what if this system we rely on, this hand that feeds us, is unknowingly nurturing a hidden danger?

There's a silent storm brewing, one called Antimicrobial Resistance (AMR). It's the terrifying reality of infections becoming untreatable, common remedies failing, because the microscopic bugs they target have learned to fight back. And the startling truth? The way we raise much of our food has become a major crossroads, a critical gatekeeper, in this global health emergency.

Imagine the sheer scale: a staggering amount, maybe over 70%, of the world's most vital antibiotics aren't used for sick people, but given to livestock. Often, it's not even about treating illness, but a routine measure to prevent disease in crowded barns or, in the past, simply to make animals grow faster. Picture it like a constant, low-level battlefield: every dose wipes out the vulnerable bacteria, leaving behind the tough guys – the resistant ones. These microscopic outlaws don't just vanish; they multiply, thrive, and eventually, can dominate.

And they travel. These resilient microbes, carrying their blueprints for resistance, become invisible hitchhikers. They can journey from the farm on the very meat, milk, and eggs we buy, surviving processing and handling to potentially end up in our homes. It's an unsettling thought – the food meant to nourish us could carry passengers that undermine the medicines meant to heal us.

It's not just life on land. Our "watery farms," the aquaculture operations bringing us fish and shellfish, face similar pressures. As we demand more seafood, these farms intensify, creating conditions where diseases – and subsequently, antibiotics – can spread like wildfire. This includes drugs crucial for human health, seeding resistance in aquatic life and the waters they inhabit. Residues of drugs might linger, but the bigger ghost at the feast is the resistant bacteria themselves, silently passing through the food chain. Even the earth isn't spared, as manure from treated animals, used as fertilizer, can lace our soils and potentially our plant-based foods with these hardy germs.

But here's where the story can pivot. If our food system is a powerful gatekeeper that's been inadvertently letting the threat through, it also holds the key to locking it out. We stand at a turning point, with the chance to reimagine how we produce food, guided by the wisdom that the health of people, animals, and our planet are deeply intertwined – the very essence of "One Health."

This isn't just wishful thinking; change is already rustling through the fields and fisheries. We're seeing the rise of food raised without routine antibiotics. This demands a smarter, more humane approach: giving animals better living conditions, strengthening their natural defenses through good welfare, using vaccines proactively, and exploring innovative allies like probiotics or bacteria-fighting viruses (phages).

Need proof it can work? Look at Denmark's pig farmers. Faced with rising resistance, they didn't throw up their hands. They changed the rules, drastically cutting antibiotic use by focusing on health, tracking everything meticulously, and working together. The result? A thriving industry and a significant drop in drug dependence. Or consider the move towards "AMR-aware" seafood. While a specific label might be new, sustainable certifications are increasingly asking tough questions about antibiotic use, demanding transparency and rewarding responsible practices. Think of organic farms, too – their entire philosophy leans on preventing sickness naturally, restricting antibiotics to only essential, rare cases, showing that a different path is viable.

Turning the tide against AMR isn't someone else's problem; it lands squarely on our collective plate. The food system isn't just a passive backdrop; it's an active arena where choices matter every single day. By championing preventative health for animals, embracing innovation, demanding transparency, and choosing food produced with care, we fortify that gate. It needs everyone: policymakers crafting sensible rules, farmers embracing change, vets guiding with wisdom, shops offering better choices, and us, the eaters, asking for food that nourishes our health as much as it satisfies our hunger.

The challenge is vast, yes. But the reward? Protecting the power of modern medicine, ensuring safer food, and safeguarding the health of generations to come. By transforming the hand that feeds us, we can help heal our future.

Weaving the World's Health Together: Why 'Playing Nice' Needs a Playbook

Imagine our planet's health – the well-being of people, the vitality of animals, the balance of the environment – isn't a collection of separate clinics, but one interconnected body. A fever in the rainforest canopy can eventually spike a temperature in a city hospital. A contaminated stream can ripple outwards, affecting livestock and landing on our dinner plates. This isn't just poetic; it's the fundamental truth of One Health.

But knowing we're all connected is like admiring the threads; it doesn't automatically weave the tapestry. For too long, our health heroes – doctors, vets, ecologists, farmers – have worked in their own worlds, like brilliant musicians playing solos in separate rooms. To create harmony, to tackle the big threats, we need a conductor, a shared musical score, a way to play together. That's what One Health governance models are: the practical blueprints, the handshakes-turned-into-action-plans, that turn shared understanding into life-saving teamwork. It's about building bridges, not just acknowledging the river between us.

Why the urgency? Look no further than the shadowy world of zoonotic diseases – those illnesses that vault the species barrier. A chilling statistic whispers that around 60-75% of new infectious diseases make this leap from animals to humans. Think avian flu, Ebola, or the next unwelcome microbial surprise lurking just out of sight. When these sparks fly, trying to douse the flames from separate fire stations – public health here, veterinary services there, wildlife experts somewhere else – is dangerously slow and clumsy. We've seen it happen: fragmented responses in the early days of outbreaks often mean lost time, wasted resources, and ultimately, a higher human cost. We need a coordinated emergency call system, not just hoping someone picks up the phone.

The global conversation is catching up. While a specific "2025 Global One Health Policy" might still be on the drawing board, the idea is electrifying discussions worldwide. Preparing for the next pandemic, building health systems that can bend without breaking – everyone agrees this requires weaving different sectors together. Researchers are constantly mapping the landscape, figuring out what makes these collaborations work. Their findings often point to essential ingredients: strong leadership that believes in the mission, dedicated money to fuel the engine, clear rules of engagement, shared 'early warning systems' for risks, and open channels for information. It's like building a team; you need trust, clear roles, and a shared game plan. Sometimes, success hinges on creating a neutral "huddle space" where different ministries, maybe used to competing, can finally talk openly and build trust.

Consider the slow-motion crisis of Antimicrobial Resistance (AMR) – the rise of superbugs. This is a perfect storm brewed in a One Health pot. Antibiotics overused in human medicine, essential drugs relied upon in farming and animal care – it all contributes. Resistant bacteria don't respect borders or species; they travel through food, water, and us. Recognizing this tangled web, many nations are now assembling AMR Task Forces. Picture them: Health, Agriculture, and Environment ministries sitting at the same table, alongside scientists and regulators. These aren't just discussion groups; they're intended as command centers, tasked with rolling out national battle plans, tracking superbugs across humans and animals, promoting smarter antibiotic use everywhere, and getting the word out to the public. But here's the key: their real power depends on the governance behind them. Do they have the clout to make changes, or are they just advisory bodies? Strong governance makes the difference between a plan on paper and genuine progress.

Want a glimpse of this in action? Look at Kenya's Zoonotic Disease Unit (ZDU). This isn't just an acronym; it's a living bridge connecting the country's human health and animal health worlds. Specifically for AMR, they've pioneered integrated surveillance. Data from doctors' clinics and vets' labs flow into a shared pool. Suddenly, you can see the bigger picture: how resistance is moving, where the hotspots are. This shared intelligence allows for smarter, targeted actions – maybe changing antibiotic guidelines in hospitals and advising farmers on livestock practices simultaneously. The Kenyan ZDU shows how a dedicated coordinating body, backed by formal agreements (the governance!), translates the One Health idea into real health protection.

And the world is full of different flavors of this approach. Germany has a platform knitting researchers together across disciplines. The US CDC's One Health Office acts as an internal coordinator within a massive government system. In Southeast Asia, regional networks foster cross-border collaboration on disease tracking. Each model is tailored to its unique context, its politics, its most pressing health threats. There's no single magic recipe, but the core ingredients – collaboration, communication, coordination – are universal.

Ultimately, designing these collaborative frameworks isn't about adding another layer of bureaucracy. It's about building a more resilient, healthier future for everyone. It's about ensuring that when the next health storm gathers, we face it together, shoulder-to-shoulder, armed with shared knowledge and a coordinated plan. Moving One Health from a beautiful concept to a powerful, everyday reality is one of the most critical tasks of our time.

About Author

Azhar ul Haque Sario is a bestselling author and data scientist with a remarkable record of achievement. This Cambridge alumnus brings a wealth of knowledge to his work, holding an MBA, ACCA (Knowledge Level - FTMS College Malaysia), BBA, and several Google certifications, including specializations in Google Data Analytics, Google Digital Marketing & E-commerce, and Google Project Management.

With ten years of business experience, Azhar combines practical expertise with his impressive academic background to craft insightful books. His prolific writing has resulted in an astounding 2810 published titles, earning him the record for the maximum Kindle editions and paperback books published by an individual author in one year, awarded by Asia Books of Records in 2024.

ORCID: https://orcid.org/0009-0004-8629-830X
Azhar.sario@hotmail.co.uk
https://www.linkedin.com/in/azharulhaquesario/

www.ingramcontent.com/pod-product-compliance
Lightning Source LLC
Chambersburg PA
CBHW031344230926
51848CB00002B/381